# Pilates plus
# Diet

For details of your nearest Body Control Pilates teacher, plus a wide range of Pilates equipment for home use, books, videos and accessories, send a stamped addressed envelope to:

Body Control Pilates®
PO Box 29061
London
WC2H 9TB
England

Or visit the Body Control Pilates® website at www.bodycontrol.co.uk

A capsule collection of comfortable, hi-performance sportswear is available to buy on the internet www.bodycontrolclothing.com.

Other Body Control Pilates® Books

Body Control the Pilates Way
0 330 36945 8 / £7.99

The Mind–Body Workout
0 330 36946 6 / £12.99

Pilates: The Way Forward
0 330 37081 2 / £12.99

The Official Body Control Pilates Manual
0 330 39327 8 / £12.99

Pilates Gym
0 330 48309 9 / £12.99

The Body Control Pilates Back Book
0 330 48311 0 / £9.99

The Body Control Pilates Pocket Traveller
0 330 49106 7 / £4.99

Intelligent Exercise with Pilates & Yoga
0 333 98952 X / £16.99

The Perfect Body the Pilates Way
0 333 90752 3 / £18.99

These titles are available from all good bookshops, or can be ordered direct from:
Book Services By Post
PO Box 29
Douglas
Isle of Man
IM99 IBQ

Credit card hotline +44 (0) 1624 677 237
Postage and packing free in the UK
or online at www.bodycontrol.co.uk
Watch out for new titles!

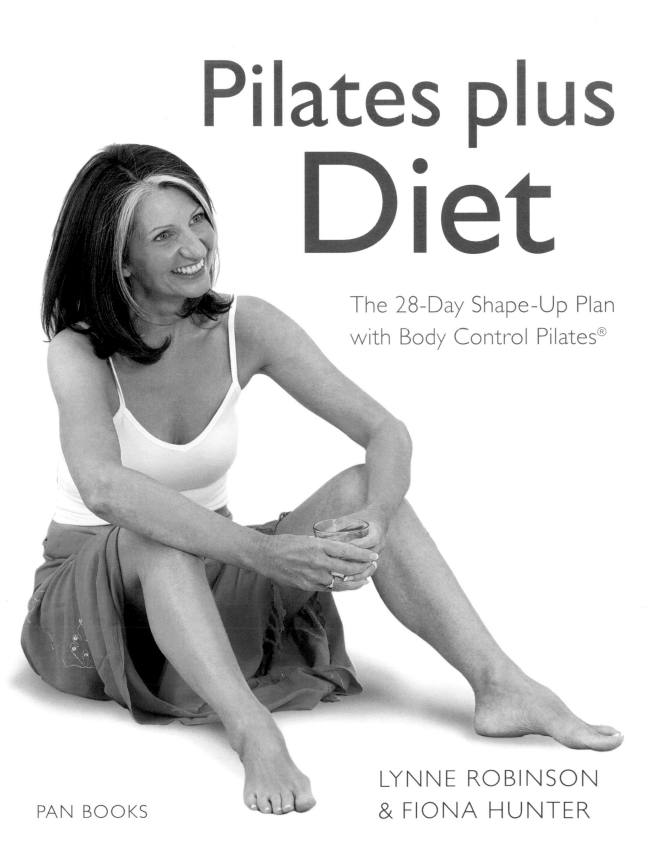

# Pilates plus Diet

## The 28-Day Shape-Up Plan with Body Control Pilates®

LYNNE ROBINSON
& FIONA HUNTER

PAN BOOKS

First published 2003 by Pan Books
an imprint of Pan Macmillan Ltd
Pan Macmillan, 20 New Wharf Road, London N1 9RR
Basingstoke and Oxford
Associated companies throughout the world
www.panmacmillan.com

ISBN  0 330 48954 2

Photography by Jim Marks
Illustrations by Raymond Turvey

9 8 7 6 5 4 3 2 1

A CIP catalogue record for this book
is available from the British Library.

Typeset by SX Composing DTPL
Printed and bound in Great Britain by Bath Press

# Contents

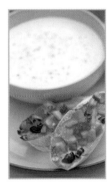
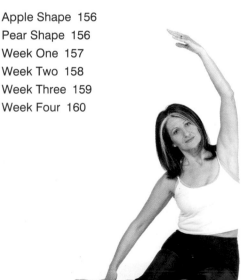

# Acknowledgements

*The Pilates Method*
*'is designed to give you suppleness,*
*natural grace and skill that will be*
*unmistakably reflected in the way*
*you walk, in the way you play,*
*and in the way you work'*

Joseph Pilates

Once again, I would like to give my thanks to everyone in the Body Control Pilates team for their continued support, enthusiasm and professionalism.

A big thank you to Fiona for agreeing to co-author this book, and to Caroline Brien for her invaluable help in this project.

Thanks to Michael Tabona and his staff at the Hotel Fortina spa resort in Sliema, Malta for having the vision to bring Body Control Pilates and Fiona's dietary approach together under one roof – a special thanks to Bryn, the Pilates Studio Director, Alan, the physiotherapist and Peter, the Head Chef.

Lynne Robinson

# How to Use This Book

The key to this programme's effectiveness is its simplicity. We have divided the book into easy-to-follow chapters so that you can clearly see the background and basics of both the Body Control Pilates and the nutritional approaches. You will find all the exercises in chapter 3 and recipes for breakfast, lunch and supper in chapter 5. Your daily meal planner plan starts on page 111. Your daily exercise workouts start on page 157. You will also find tips and advice to keep you directed and motivated.

The exercises are clearly explained and then combined in five 30-minute workouts for four weeks. Each workout is different, yet perfectly balanced and can be done at home with no expensive equipment. You just need to add three 20-minute plus aerobic workouts a week to your routine.

If you don't exercise or eat properly one day, don't dwell on it but move on. Above all, we want you to enjoy using this book, so take time to read it and you and your body will really get the most out if it!

## Before You Begin

Equipment you will need:
- A padded, non-slip mat.
- A folded towel or small, flat cushion.
- A plump cushion.
- A pillow.
- A tennis ball.
- A scarf, long towel or stretch band.
- Loose, comfortable clothing and bare feet.
- Hand-held weights of up to about 2.5kg each weight, or easily held household items of the same weight. (You may use heavier weights if you wish to 'sculpt' the arms.)
- Ankle weights of up to about 1kg each weight. Alternatively, use a pair of old tights (no holes!) – cut off the legs, tie a knot about 15 centimetres from the end, pour in uncooked rice and then tie a knot about 15 centimetres from the other end. Repeat with the other leg and wrap around your ankles as needed.

Please do not exercise if:
- You are feeling unwell.
- You have just eaten a heavy meal.
- You have been drinking alcohol.
- You are in pain from an injury. Consult your practitioner first.
- You have been taking painkillers because they will mask any warning signs.
- You are undergoing medical treatment or are taking drugs. Consult your practitioner first.

It is always wise to consult your doctor before taking up a new exercise regime. Many of the exercises are wonderful for back-related problems, but you should seek expert guidance.

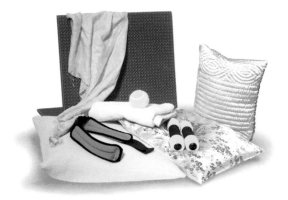

# The Balanced Approach to a Healthy Body

It's no secret that diet and exercise work hand in hand to achieve or maintain a healthy body. Yet even in our information-rich world, many people still prefer to eat less than is good for them in order to stay slim or eat the wrong foods after a workout. Presented with so many choices in health and fitness – which diet? which exercise? – it's no wonder many of us are confused.

This book gives you a simple 28-day programme of nutritious meals and effective exercises that will enable you to achieve your goals of better health and a better body using a common-sense approach. It is a self-help guide to total health and fitness, increased vitality and lasting weight control. It will boost your energy, improve your cardio health and your immune system and enhance the shape, tone and flexibility of your body. Used properly, the next 28 days will change your life and your shape forever. Even better, you will start to notice and feel the results within a short time.

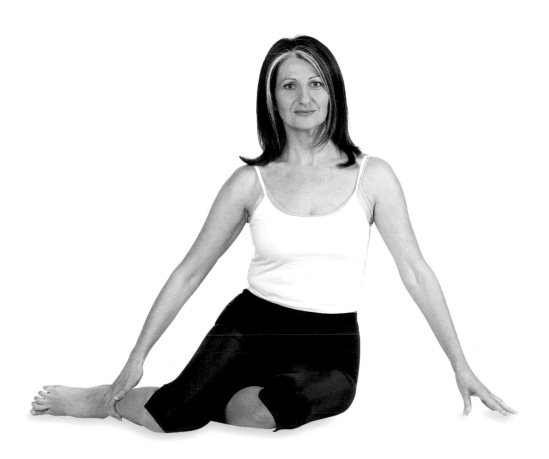

## Never Say Never

Perhaps you think it's too late to change, that you are stuck with your body the way it is. Definitely not! Your whole body is being continually renewed, mainly through the proteins you eat, and about 98 per cent of your body's molecules, including muscles, bones, teeth and organs, are totally rebuilt each year.

In fact . . .
- Your skin is just one month old.
- Your blood Is about three months old.
- The protein in your muscle is less than six months old.

This programme will change you at a cellular level, inside and out. Your hair, eyes, skin, nails, bones, muscles, organs and all the body's systems – circulatory, respiratory, lymphatic, digestive – will be affected by it. That's why we can promise that if you follow it, you will see real results at the end of 28 days. We also hope you will be so happy with the new you that you will want to continue with this way of eating and exercising.

## The Secrets of Success

We are all trying to find the secret of eternal youth. Some of us resort to cosmetic surgery, even though these procedures can carry health risks. We do this because it's a quick fix: you opt for liposuction because you think the alternative is hours sweating at the gym and eating nothing but cabbage. But this isn't true. One look at the delicious recipes in this book should be enough to convince anyone that healthy eating isn't boring eating. And five 30-minute sessions of Pilates body conditioning, plus three 20-minute aerobic sessions a week is not that demanding. As you build more muscle your metabolic rate changes and remains elevated even after your workout, so you continue to burn calories even when resting. Add this to the other benefits of this programme and you won't feel the need of the surgeon's knife.

Following the 28-day programme and adopting this new healthy lifestyle will:
- reduce the risk of heart disease, hypertension and high cholesterol
- prevent and reverse osteoporosis and osteoarthritis
- flatten your stomach, tone your thighs and trim your hips
- redefine your waist
- streamline and reshape your body
- minimize cellulite by improving circulation and drainage and by toning your muscles
- give you legs to die for
- reduce stress and anxiety
- increase your sense of vitality and wellbeing
- condition both your mind and your body
- improve your posture
- reduce back pain
- increase flexibility
- give you a long lean look
- give you unlimited energy
- improve your immunity
- reverse many signs of ageing
- boost your self-confidence and self-esteem

Of course, there is the added advantage that this programme will help you lose body fat which alone, although it isn't easy, gives enormous health benefits. Many experts believe that the real reason for the alarming rise in levels of obesity witnessed over the last decade is not because we eat more, but because we do less.

An increasing amount of our free time is spent watching television, playing computer games or surfing the net. Modern technology and labour-saving devices mean that we're much less active than we used to be. The average amount of time spent watching television has doubled to 27 hours a week in just 30 years.

*'It is the spirit itself which shapes the body'*

Joseph Pilates

If you've ever watched the calories slowly burning off while you furiously pedal away on an exercise bike, you'll already know that exercise alone is not a very efficient way of getting rid of excess weight. But exercise does play a very important role in dieting. If you exercise at the same time as dieting, more of the weight you lose will be fat rather than lean muscle tissue. Exercise preserves and develops muscle tissue which is metabolically more active than fat (it uses up more calories than fat). In other words, the more muscle you have the more calories your body burns, not just while you are exercising, but when you are going about your daily activities and even while you are sleeping. Pilates exercises can therefore help to change your metabolic rate. Uniquely challenging yet deceptively simple, they offer a clear logical programme to take you step by step towards that stronger, more supple, leaner body and better health.

The basic message of our programme is very simple – a healthy balanced diet combined with the right type of exercises can change your shape permanently and improve your overall wellbeing, offering you boundless energy and endless vitality and keeping you looking and feeling youthful.

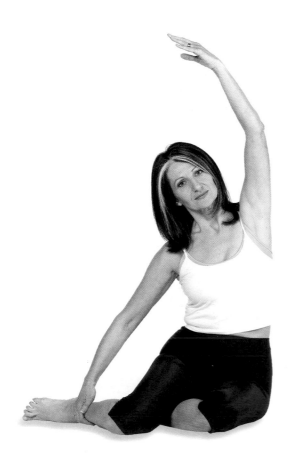

# Building Strength from Within

One of the most important aims of this book is to convince you to set aside the idea that the weight of your body is the best indicator of physical fitness. A far better guide to levels of fitness is, in fact, an analysis of your body composition. Body composition refers to the amount of lean and fat tissue that make up your total body weight. Lean tissue comprises muscle, organs, bone and water. Wild animals have a high percentage of lean body mass, which gives them their stamina and their powerful, streamlined graceful bodies.

*'Read through the whole exercise; imagine it in your mind. Visualizing it will help you do it'*

Lynne Robinson

Central to our programme therefore is the creation of a lean and muscular body. This doesn't mean you will become less feminine or develop bulky muscles because we will be building strength from within. What it does mean is eating a healthy balanced diet and taking the right kind of exercise. We recommend Pilates exercises because they teach good movement skills, body awareness, good postural alignment, efficient breathing and core stability. We have included Pilates exercises for strength training in the programme, using free weights and gravity resistance to increase your lean body mass by building muscle. In addition, we recommend you take part in regular aerobic activity to improve your cardiovascular health which strengthens the heart and lungs and enhances your body's ability to transport oxygen which is needed by the body to enable you to burn calories and fat.

Joseph Pilates said that his exercises were 'designed to give you suppleness, natural grace and skill that will be unmistakably reflected in the way you walk, in the way you play and in the way you work. You will develop muscular power with corresponding endurance, ability to perform arduous duties, to play strenuous games, to walk, run or travel for long distances without undue body fatigue or mental strain.'

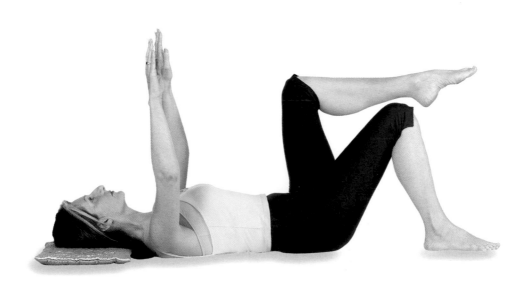

# The Energy Balance Equation

There is no mystery as to why we gain weight, it's a simple equation: we gain weight when the energy (calories) that we consume exceeds the energy (calories) we use and excess energy (calories) is therefore stored in the body as fat. Eating just a small amount in excess of your needs will result in a slow but steady weight gain. Eating 100 calories a day more than you need – the equivalent of 1½ digestive biscuits – will result in weight gain of 4.7kg in a year. But the long-term answer to weight control is not simply a case of calorie counting. Without doubt it is part of it, but the best way to control your weight is by a combination of the right diet and the right type of exercise.

*'What is balance of body and mind? It is the conscious control of all muscular movements of the body'*

Joseph Pilates

## Body Weight Versus Body Fat

The scales never lie, but they can distort the truth! It is quite possible for someone to be within the ideal weight range, as determined by a weight-for-height chart, yet still to be carrying too much fat. Equally, because muscle is heavier than fat, a very muscular person may appear overweight when judged by the same chart. Your body composition – that is how much of your weight is fat and where that fat is stored – is an important factor in determining the health risks associated with being overweight.

Your total weight is far less relevant than the proportion of lean tissue to fat, which needs to be within established recommended limits if you wish to avoid the many health problems associated with being overweight such as high blood pressure, high cholesterol levels, arteriosclerosis, coronary disease and respiratory disorders. We must also not forget the dangers of having too little body fat, and the dangers of anorexia nervosa or bulimia.

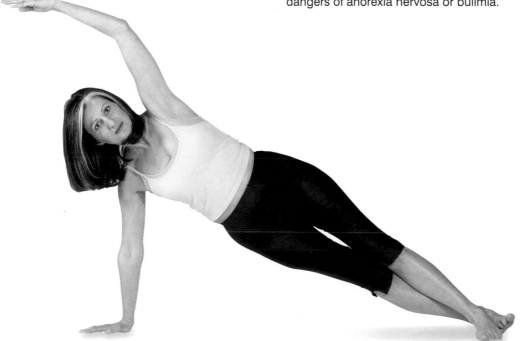

## Apples and Pears

Fat stored round the waist, producing an apple-shaped body, is more likely to be linked with health problems particularly an increased risk of non-insulin diabetes, heart disease, high blood pressure and abnormal blood fat levels. In women, central obesity is associated with a higher risk of pre-menopausal breast cancer. Fat stored around the hips in a pear shape seems to be less problematic.

Whether you are an 'apple' or a 'pear' is partly an inherited tendency influenced by your genetic make-up. However, certain factors such as smoking and drinking alcohol seem to increase the likelihood of fat being laid down in the stomach area, while exercise helps reduce stomach fat. There is some evidence to suggest that it's easier to lose central fat than that stored around the hips.

As discussed earlier, our bodies are made up of two components: lean body mass (LBM) and fat. Lean body mass consists of organs such as the heart, the liver and the pancreas, and bones and skin and, of course, muscle tissue. All of these need oxygen and nutrients from food for growth, renewal and repair. Muscle, in particular, has a high metabolic rate and burns calories quickly. Lean body mass is constantly altering because of changes in your muscles. The rest of your body is made up of fat which does not need oxygen, doesn't repair itself and has a low metabolic rate, so it doesn't burn calories.

People who have a low lean body mass are usually lacking in energy, and studies have shown that they are as much at risk from degeneration and premature ageing as people who have too much body fat. It is the ratio of lean body mass to fat and the distribution of that fat that determines the health risks associated with being overweight. The problem with many slimming and detox diets is that they result in shedding muscle rather than fat. If you rely on faddish diets to keep you slim and ignore exercise, your body will gradually lose tone, you'll lose lean muscle tissue, your energy levels will become depleted and your overall health will be affected.

If you want to streamline your body permanently, improve the condition of your hair, skin and bones, improve your energy levels, boost your immune system and achieve optimum health, you need to increase your lean body mass through correct diet and the right exercise. For a typical adult man, an average body fat percentage would be 15–20 per cent (if overweight it would be over 25 per cent and if obese over 30 per cent). For a typical adult woman, average body fat is 25–27 per cent (if overweight it would be over 30 per cent and if obese over 35 per cent).

# Measuring Total Body Fat

There are several methods by which total body fat can be measured. The most accurate are complicated, expensive and used only in specialist research centres. Measuring body fat can be a useful way to monitor the progress of a diet programme, which incorporates exercise as well as calorie restriction (as all the best ones should). As muscle is heavier than fat, if fat is lost but replaced by muscle, ordinary scales may fail to register any weight loss. In practice, when people are exercising they can feel their bodies becoming firmer, fitter and better toned as fat is replaced by muscle but sometimes it is nice to have those feelings confirmed. So while body weight is not always a good indicator of body fat, for most of us it's still a useful way of finding out if we need to lose weight.

Body Mass Index (BMI) is a more accurate predictor of the health risks associated with being overweight than weight alone. There is a wealth of scientific evidence that suggests a BMI between 18.5 and 25 is associated with the lowest heath risks; the risks increase slightly below 18.5, increase significantly above 25 and increase dramatically with a BMI over 30. Although BMI doesn't give you information about body fat, using it in conjunction with waist circumference will give you a better idea. If your BMI is above 25 and your waist circumference is above 80 centimetres for a woman and 94 centimetres for a man, it suggests that the excess weight you're carrying is fat and not muscle.

# Measuring Fat

A growing number of health clubs, spas and doctors' surgeries will now measure body fat as well as body weight. The results are unlikely to be 100 per cent accurate and vary slightly depending on the method used, but they can give you a useful idea of your total body fat. Since the distribution of body fat is just as important as the amount, it is also worth measuring waist circumference. For this you need nothing more sophisticated than a tape measure! If you are interested in monitoring the change in your body fat over a period of time, in the comfort of your own home, you might like to invest in a Body Fat Analyser. It looks like a set of regular bathroom scales and will measure weight in the usual way, but at the same time it will also measure body fat.

## How You Shape Up

You can work out your BMI using this simple equation:
BMI = your weight (in kilos) ÷ your height (in meters) squared
e.g.: 60kg ÷ (1.65mx1.65m) = 22

1kg = 2.2 lbs     1m = 39.37 inches

18.5-25  is acceptable
25-30  overweight
30-40  obese
over 40  severely obese

## Percentage of Body Fat

You need to lose weight if your percentage of body fat is:
over 33 per cent for women
over 25 per cent for men

# 1

## The Building Blocks of the
## **Pilates Plus Diet** Programme

# The Building Blocks of a Balanced Fitness Programme

Even if you follow the healthiest, most balanced diet available and take all the latest nutritional supplements on the shelves, it won't make up for lack of exercise. Our bodies are designed to move.

The question is which type of exercise is best for achieving lasting weight control, total fitness and overall wellbeing? If your primary goal is permanent fat loss, you need to choose exercise that is effective, slow and sustained, that will increase your metabolism, improve your ratio of lean body mass to fat and increase your supply of oxygen to the muscle cells. Does one exercise provide all this? The truthful answer is no.

Pilates can provide almost all of your needs because it is, in essence, an interdisciplinary method. What most people don't realize is that Pilates has elements from many different types of fitness and movement training. If you watch a Pilates class in action, whether it is a mat class or a studio session with machinery, you will see exercises similar to classical ballet training but we also use both free weights and resistance training. You will also notice movements that remind you of the martial arts and yoga. This is because Joseph Pilates drew from all these fitness techniques when building his own exercise programme during the 1920s. Underlying every exercise was an awareness of moving well, retraining and re-educating your body. If you are looking for a complete fitness programme then Pilates can provide you with everything you need, except cardiovascular work, so you will need to add aerobic activity to your schedule.

So what are the basic ingredients of our programme?

- good movement skills – the basis of Body Control Pilates
- joint mobility exercises
- flexibility training
- strength training
- aerobic activity

# Good Movement Skills

Let's take a brief look at how movement takes place. Bones go nowhere by themselves, they need muscles to move them.

The muscles themselves need instructions, so we must consider the 'control' or the 'intelligent' part of the system: the nervous system. Muscle is controlled by the nervous system, which sends electrochemical energy impulses to the muscle fibres signalling them to contract which, in turn, makes the bones move. There is also a constant sensory feedback to the brain – your pro-prioception – which tells the brain what's happening, where your body is in space, how it's moving, and so on. There is therefore a constant flow of messages to and from the brain, constant input and output.

What is starting to come to the fore in medical research is the importance of good input. In other words, the brain remembers how you are moving. It remembers patterns of movement – good or bad. Unfortunately most of us move badly. We no longer perform the wide range of activities our bodies were originally designed for – running, skipping, jumping and climbing. Instead, we spend far too much time sitting (and sitting badly for that matter), and our activities tend to be repetitive day in, day out.

> *'When standing, remember that the three main body weights – the head, the ribcage and the pelvis – should be balanced centrally over each other'*
> Lynne Robinson

This affects both the length and strength of our muscles and their functions, and may ultimately bring the body out of good postural alignment, placing stress on our joints. Bad input equals bad output. What the Pilates Method does is use simple exercises performed with awareness and control to reprogramme your body. Good input equals good output. If the brain receives the right messages (by repeating good movements during Pilates exercises) these messages will be locked into your muscle memory banks! Joseph Pilates recognized this when he repeated his favourite quote from Schiller, 'It is the mind itself which builds the body.'

We cannot stress enough the importance of learning to move with awareness, good alignment and core stability (see chapter 2). Otherwise you are merely reinforcing bad movements and adding more stress and strain to your joints. This is why you must practice the exercises in the section called The Basics of Body Control Pilates (pages 37–50) before you attempt the main programme. This will give you the essential skills you need to continue the learning process with the recommended workouts.

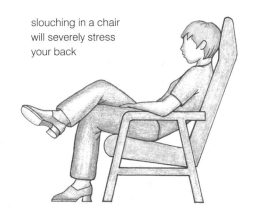

sitting correctly greatly reduces the pressure on the discs

slouching in a chair will severely stress your back

# Joint Mobility Exercises

A joint is simply where two bones meet. There are many factors involved in the health of a joint but one of the main ones is correct alignment. Let's look at the hip joint.

The head of the femur, or thigh bone, is designed to sit snugly in the acetabulum, or hip socket. The idea is that the two fit perfectly together, bathed by synovial fluid which keeps both surfaces well oiled when movement takes place. If, because of poor posture and muscle imbalance, the joint is held out of alignment, then the forces of gravity will no longer fall through the centre of the joint and there is going to be unnecessary wear and tear on the surfaces, less lubrication and the potential for arthritis or injury.

Different joints have different movement potential according to their structure. We therefore need to bear in mind which movements are suitable for which joints in order to work within the body's natural range of motion. If you stress a joint by forcing or twisting it in a direction that is unnatural, you risk weakening or injuring that joint.

With the hip joint, for example, we should be able to make the following movements:

If we lose the ability to make these movements easily, we compromise not only the health of the hip joint itself but our whole body's movement. With hip replacement operations reaching epidemic proportions, clearly we are doing something wrong!

The keys to healthy joints are:

- Good overall health.
- Good postural alignment ensuring joints are held naturally in their ideal neutral alignment. The joints should be supported by strong stabilizing muscles and ligaments holding the bones in good alignment and allowing free-flowing movement to take place.
- Exercise that takes the joints through their full range of movement and which encourages lubrication – the production of synovial fluid, which washes over and lubricates the joint keeping it healthy, a bit like WD40! A simple exercise such as Single Leg Circles on page 56 will help towards this goal. Spine Curls will even work on the joints in your spine (page 52).
- A healthy balanced diet – rich in essential fatty acids, especially the omega-3 marine nutrients including EPA and DHA (found in cod liver oil).

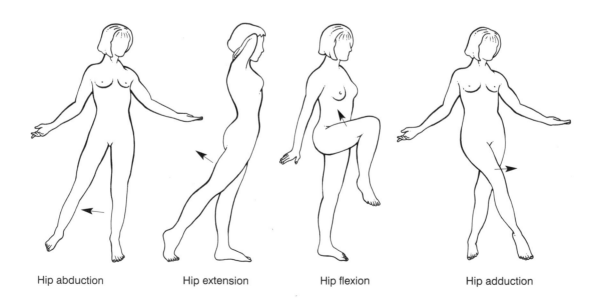

Hip abduction          Hip extension          Hip flexion          Hip adduction

# Flexibility Training

Stretching feels great and is an essential part of any fitness programme, hence the popularity of stretch classes. We are aiming for bodies that are both flexible and strong. Flexibility is a very individual thing. Some of us are born supple – when you were at school some children could easily do the splits or a backward bend, while others struggled. Nothing is more frustrating than working out next to a dancer who effortlessly places her forehead on her knee in a forward bend while you are having difficulty moving a mere few centimetres forward from the vertical plane! But you must bear in mind that a variety of factors are going to influence how flexible you are and many of them are out of your control. Above all, stretching should never be competitive.

Factors that may influence your flexibility include:
- the structure and health of the joint
- the restriction of movement by surrounding muscles and connective tissue
- the temperature of the joint and surrounding tissues
- the elasticity of your muscle tissue
- the presence of scar tissue
- the elasticity of your tendons and ligaments
- the elasticity of your skin
- your age
- your gender (females tend to be more flexible)
- the outside temperature
- the time of day
- past injury
- your mental approach – can you relax?

There are different types of stretching techniques available. In this programme we will be using dynamic and static stretches.

**Dynamic Stretching**

Recent studies have shown the importance of dynamic stretching (also called active extensions) which is the type of flexibility work Joseph Pilates primarily used. Dynamic stretching occurs as part of a movement where you use the opposing muscle to stretch another muscle. The beauty of dynamic stretching is that it is a totally natural way to achieve flexibility and there is little chance of over-stretching.

For example, in the Double Leg Stretch (page 68), as the legs are extended the quadriceps (at the front of the thighs ) work to stretch the hamstrings (at the back of the thighs).

## Static Stretching

There are two types of static stretching: active, where you maintain an extended position with just the strength of the muscles, for example, holding a leg out to the side; and passive, where you use gravity or some piece of apparatus to maintain a position as in the Studio Adductor Stretch on page 53.

Traditionally, stretching has been used for different purposes:

* Warm up: stretching can play a valuable role as part of a warm up for many activities. You may use the gentle passive static stretches for this, for example the Beachball Hamstring Stretch (page 54).
* Wind down: stretching at the end of an aerobic or strength-training session is a useful way to balance the muscles and reduce the accumulation of lactic acid, which is a by-product of vigorous exercise causing the burning sensation you sometimes feel after a strenuous workout and which can lead to muscle stiffness.
* Both active static and dynamic stretches can be used. Arm Openings on page 82 is a good dynamic wind-down stretch.

## Developmental Stretching

Flexibility may be increased by developmental stretching. We are aiming here for a more permanent change in muscle length, so the stretches will be held for longer and will be more challenging. For this type of stretching it is crucial that the body be thoroughly warmed up, so developmental stretching is ideal after an aerobic session. If you wish to achieve a developmental stretch, use a passive static stretch.

## Guidelines for Stretches

* Clothes should be comfortable and warm and should not restrict your movements.
* Always ensure that your muscles are warm before they are stretched. Tissue is more pliable when warm. You will notice that we place the stretches at a point in your workout where you should be nicely warmed up.
* Check your alignment constantly. In stretching, joints normally, but not always, remain in neutral (page 39) to prevent stress and to ensure that you isolate the right muscle.
* Be aware of any tension creeping into other parts of the body, especially the neck, jaw, shoulders, calves, feet and hands.
* Use your breathing to help. Initiate the stretch on the out breath, stabilize, and then breathe normally during the stretch, relaxing into it (page 38).
* Start the stretch easily, then if you can stretch a little further this brings you to the developmental part of the stretch. Allow the muscle to lengthen.
* For a developmental stretch you need to allow time for the stretch to happen. We suggest 20 to 30 seconds, but it may take longer for the muscle to lengthen and release.
* Never bounce in a stretch or stretch to the point of pain, as this only brings in a mechanism known as the 'stretch reflex' which is when a nerve reflex responds by signalling the muscle to contract in order to prevent the muscle from being injured.
* Although you will be relaxing into the stretch you should always remain in control.
* Recover slowly from a stretch, remembering all your good movement principles.
* A stretch should never be painful, you should feel it but it should remain a pleasant experience. Any tension should be felt in the muscle itself.
* Be prepared for your body to change from one day to the next.
* Above all, enjoy the stretch. If you are not enjoying it, you're not doing it right!

# Strength Training

Aerobic activity strengthens the heart and lungs while weight training has the following benefits:

- It strengthens the joints and the muscles supporting the joints.
- It increases muscle mass, improving the lean body mass to fat ratio (page 12).

It also prevents and helps reverse osteoporosis. About 30 per cent of women and 5 per cent of men will suffer from osteoporosis or brittle bone disease which is defined as a loss of bone mineral leading to thinning of the bone. Although bone looks very solid, it is in fact full of holes rather like coral. Bone health is determined by nutrition, by mineral and vitamin content and by the amount of stress it is put under. This is one type of stress that is good for us! Bones are thicker and stronger when they are stressed, because stress produces electrical effects in the bone that encourage bone growth. If there is no stress, the bone will be less dense and weaker. During our lives there is a constant turnover of bone – up to the age of thirty-five we lose as much old bone each year as we make new bone, so there is no problem. From thirty-five on, however, we tend to lose about 1 per cent of our bone mass each year until we reach menopause when bone loss accelerates with a further loss of 2 per cent per year for up to ten years. By the age of seventy, approximately one third of bone mass will be lost.

Bone mass is affected by:

- Hormonal status: menopausal women in particular have an accelerated bone loss, which comes with the decline in production of the amount of the ovarian hormone oestrogen.
- Diet: especially the inclusion of naturally occurring plant oestrogens and calcium in our diet during our growing years.
- Genetic factors: which determine the size of our bones and muscles.
- Physical activity: particularly weight-bearing exercise.

Recent research has shown that regular weight-bearing exercise can help prevent the onset of osteoporosis and the earlier we start weight training the better – even in our teens we can be laying good foundations for the future.

Until very recently, weight training received much bad press. People have associated it with serious bodybuilding and, although this has its merits, the popular image of muscle-bound 'pumped-up' men and women does not appeal to most of us. But, as we have seen, there are many sound reasons for including some weight training in your fitness programme. Joseph Pilates suffered many health problems as a child and saw the benefits of bodybuilding and used the techniques to rebuild his own strength to the extent that he was used as a model for anatomical charts.

In this programme we will be using the following weight-training techniques:

## Free Weights

We will be using hand-held weights and ankle weights. Learn how to do the exercises first without weights to perfect your technique and then start with a light weight, about 0.5kg each, for both hand and leg weights. Slowly increase the weight. There is no restriction on the weight for the hands, it depends on personal choice, but you must be able to do the exercise correctly without strain or loss of technique. You should be able to lift a weight at least eight times. If you can't, it is too heavy and you would be better to do more repetitions with a lighter weight. Ankle weights of up to a maximum of 1.25kg each weight are recommended. The last repetition of a weight exercise should feel difficult.

Do not use weights targeting the same body parts more than three times a week and leave a day between weight-training sessions. When you use a weight, you actually break down muscle tissue, causing very small tears in it. Between 24 and 48 hours later, the body responds to these tears by building new muscle. But you can overuse muscles, which will set you back rather than move you on. We have planned for this in your workout schedules.

## Gravity Resistance

The other type of weight-bearing exercises we use to build strength are gravity resistant ones. This is great for any self-help programme because no special equipment is needed. Exercises such as Front Leg Pull (page 78), and even simple Curl Ups (page 58), use the body's own weight against gravity to build strength.

Whichever weight training you decide to do, exercise before you eat because it helps burn fat quickly.

Other types of weight training you could consider, but which are beyond the scope of this book are:

- Pilates Studio workout: Joseph Pilates was a natural genius for developing specialized equipment to help his clients achieve the strength and flexibility they needed to perform his classical full mat programme. The machines you find in Pilates studios today have hardly changed at all from those originals and still use spring resistance. You can now buy good home-use equipment (see page 2).
- The toning circle: this is also known by several other names but is a useful piece of portable equipment common in Pilates studios. It is essentially a lightweight steel circle that you squeeze with various parts of the body. This has to be a girl's best friend when it comes to toning the inner thighs and upper arms (see page 2).
- Resistance or stretch bands: thick bands of rubber with varying strengths (indicated by the different colours), which can be used for a variety of resistance work. Great to pop in a suitcase (see page 2).
- Gym machines: the type of weight machines you find in gyms can be useful for building muscle, but you must have good movement, core stability and awareness skills before you use them. They can limit your range of motion somewhat and it is very easy to misuse the body while exercising with them. If you decide to add gym work to your schedule, invest in a personal trainer (ideally one who is also qualified in Pilates), and read *Pilates Gym – The Balanced Workout* by Robinson and Convy.
- Water resistance: last, but by no means least, you can use water as natural resistance. There are many aqua classes to choose from which are fun to do and gentle on arthritic joints. You can also try walking in water (that's in, not on!) at some gyms.

# Aerobic Exercise

Pilates offers you the best body-conditioning method there is, however, unless you are very advanced and can complete the Full Mat Programe, it does not include cardiovascular work, so you need to add this to your programme.

In the UK every year over 100,000 people die from heart-related illnesses. In order to improve cardiovascular efficiency, you must have a programme of aerobic exercise. Aerobic exercise also lowers cholesterol. As our cardiovascular system keeps us alive, a justification for enhancing its efficiency should not be necessary, but did you know that aerobic exercise also stimulates the oxygen supply and is thus an essential part of your fat-burning programme not just while you are exercising, but afterwards as well?

Aerobic activity improves your body's ability to transport oxygen. We have already discussed the fact that the body's fat tissues have a very low metabolic rate: they do not burn calories, only muscle cells do this. Therefore, the more muscle tissue you have, the better you will burn calories. However, you need oxygen to do this – the more oxygen your muscles receive via the bloodstream the more calories and fat you will burn.

If the thought of sweating it out alongside leotard divas fills you with horror, the good news is that any aerobic activity will do. You can choose from:

* brisk/power walking
* jogging (treadmill or outdoor)
* swimming
* cycling (stationary or outdoor)
* rollerblading
* trampolining
* spinning (instructor-led class)
* kick-boxing
* dancing
* skiing
* aerobics class
* cross trainer (machine)
* rowing (indoor or outdoor)

Most of these are fun to do, and you will feel tremendous afterwards because aerobic activity produces natural opiates and noradrenaline, a brain chemical responsible for the feel-good factor after exercise.

General guidelines for aerobic exercise are:

* Have a check-up with a doctor before embarking on any exercise programme.
* Choose an activity or class to suit your level of fitness, physical limitations and needs. Find out as much information as you can by reading and talking to qualified and experienced people.
* Use a heart-rate monitor where possible (they are very easy to use). Exercising at the correct intensity is essential to ensure safe and effective training.
* Do not go too fast too soon. Build your fitness steadily and progressively and work at your own level. If you have a low level of aerobic fitness, start with moderate exercise such as walking, stationary cycling or swimming, for example.
* Exercise aerobically for a minimum of 20 minutes three to five times a week. As your aerobic fitness improves, increase the duration and intensity of your training while still monitoring your heart rate.
* Avoid carrying unnecessary tension, especially in your shoulders. Relax and monitor your breathing.
* Allow your body to rest. Have at least two days off from exercise per week. There is a fine line between training and over-training.
* Ensure that you are wearing the correct footwear especially when you are running. Incorrect footwear can lead to conditions such as shin splints and ankle injuries.

# The Building Blocks of a Balanced Diet

There is no longer any doubt that the food we eat can have an important and lasting effect on our health and wellbeing. A healthy diet can protect us against illnesses such as heart disease and cancer; it can increase resistance to colds and other infections, boost energy levels, help us cope better with the stresses and strains of modern living and improve physical and mental performance.

There are four key ingredients to a healthy diet: variety, moderation, balance and enjoyment. We need over forty different nutrients to ensure we stay fit and healthy and no single food or food group provides all the nutrients that the body needs. This is why it is important to eat a variety of foods taken from each of the five groups explained on the following pages.

Choosing a healthy diet does not have to mean saying goodbye to the foods you enjoy. A recent study found that there is a relationship between how much we enjoy our food and the nutrients we absorb from it. Eaten in moderation, there is plenty of room for all your favourites.

So what is the right balance in a healthy diet? The illustration below gives a rough guide to the balance of nutrients you should aim for over the course of a typical day.

Foods containing fats and /or sugars 8%

Meat, fish and protein-rich foods 12%

Grains, cereals, potatoes 33%

Dairy products 15%

Fruit and vegetables 33%

## Grains, Cereals, Potatoes

This food group includes bread, rice, pasta, noodles and breakfast cereals, i.e. complex or starchy carbohydrates. Nutritionists recommend that these foods should provide around one third of our calories each day. Complex carbohydrates provide dietary fibre, protein, vitamins and minerals, but their main job is to provide energy. Choose fibre-rich varieties of these foods, such as wholemeal bread and wholegrain cereals whenever possible – they provide slow-release energy which helps keep blood-sugar levels stable. High-fibre foods are more filling than their fibre-depleted counterparts, which means they help you feel full more quickly and stop you from feeling hungry for longer. Although many people still believe that foods from this group are fattening, this is only true when they are eaten with lots of fat – a rich creamy sauce with pasta, potatoes fried in fat, or bread spread thickly with butter are all highly calorific.

Depending on your appetite and calorie requirement, aim to eat between six and eleven servings from this group each day. One serving equals:
- 3 tbsp breakfast cereal
- 1 slice bread
- 2 heaped tbsp boiled rice
- 3 heaped tbsp pasta
- 2 egg-sized potatoes

# Fruit and Vegetables

It's no coincidence that in Mediterranean countries like Greece and Italy, particularly southern Italy, where people eat almost twice the amount of fruit and vegetables we do, they live longer and remain healthier. Fruit and vegetables provide vitamins and minerals, dietary fibre and phytochemicals which help protect against certain diseases. In fact, the World Cancer Research Fund estimates that a diet rich in a variety of fruit and vegetables could prevent 20 per cent of all cancers. No one fruit or vegetable can provide all the vitamins or phytochemicals you need to stay healthy, so it's important to eat a selection in order to get the variety of nutrients you need. Apart from being excellent providers of vitamins and minerals, most fruit and vegetables are fat free and wonderfully low in calories. Make the most of them – don't stick to the same old favourites but be adventurous and regularly try something new. Look for new recipes and ideas on how to cook them: try poaching, baking or grilling fruits as an alternative to eating them raw.

Aim to eat at least five servings of fruit and /or vegetables a day. Frozen, canned and dried fruits and vegetables as well as juices are useful in helping you reach that target. One serving equals:

- a small glass (150ml) unsweetened fruit juice
- 1 slice (100g) melon or pineapple
- 1 apple, orange, peach or pear
- 2 kiwi fruits, plums, satsumas or apricots
- 1 cup (100g) strawberries, raspberries or grapes
- 1 tbsp dried fruits e.g. raisins
- 3 tbsp fruit salad or cooked or canned fruit
- 2 tbsp (90g) cooked vegetables
- large bowl salad

# Dairy Products

Dairy products, including milk, cheese and yoghurt, are an important source of calcium – essential for strong bones and teeth. Many people, especially teenage girls, fail to eat enough calcium to meet their recommended daily requirement, putting themselves at risk of osteoporosis in later life. Dairy foods also provide protein, vitamin A, phosphorus, vitamin D and vitamin B2. Foods in this group can be high in fat, particularly saturated fat, so choose reduced-fat and low-fat alternatives such as skimmed and semi-skimmed milk. Calcium is contained in the non-creamy portion of milk, so when the fat is removed to make reduced-fat products the calcium remains. Pint for pint, skimmed milk contains slightly more calcium than whole milk.

Aim to eat between two and three servings from this group a day. Choose low- and reduced-fat varieties whenever possible. One serving equals:

- 1 glass of milk
- 150g carton of yoghurt
- 40g hard full-fat cheese such as Cheddar

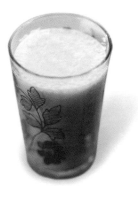

## Meat, Fish and Other Protein-rich Foods

Foods from this group provide protein which is essential for growth and development in children, for maintenance and repair of cells in adults and for the production of enzymes, antibodies and hormones. In short, protein is vital in ensuring our bodies function properly. Good sources of protein include meat, fish, eggs, cheese, beans and pulses, nuts and seeds.

If you choose meat, make sure it is lean and trim away any visible fat before cooking. Eat at least two portions of fish a week one of which should be oil-rich, such as salmon, mackerel and tuna, because they contain a large amount of omega-3 fatty acids which can help reduce the risk of heart disease and strokes by reducing cholesterol levels in the blood and making the blood less sticky and less likely to clot. Omega-3 fatty acids are also important for the health of the joints and can help ease pain associated with arthritis and are useful in treating problems like the skin condition psoriasis.

Aim to eat between two and four servings from this group a day. One serving equals approximately:
- 90g cooked red meat
- 125g chicken
- 125–150g fish
- 5 tbsp baked beans
- 2 tbsp nuts
- 2 eggs

## Foods Containing Fats and/or Sugars

Small amounts of fat are necessary in our diet to provide essential fatty acids and to allow the absorption of fat-soluble vitamins. However a high-fat diet is known to increase the risk of heart disease, certain types of cancer and obesity. A diet that is rich in saturated fats – found in foods such as fatty cuts of meats, full-fat dairy products, butter and some types of margarine – increases the levels of cholesterol in the blood which can clog the blood vessels restricting the flow of blood to the heart and increasing the risk of heart disease and stroke. Weight for weight, fat provides twice as many calories as carbohydrate or protein and there is some evidence to suggest that calories eaten as fat are more likely to be stored as body fat than calories from protein or carbohydrate. These days, low-fat does not have to mean low taste. There are easy ways to trim fat from your diet without giving up the foods you enjoy.

Sugar contains 'empty' calories that provide nothing else in the way of protein, fibre, vitamins or minerals – just calories – so it makes sense to cut down on sugar where you can. But it isn't necessary to cut it out completely: research carried out by Trinity College in Ireland found that people were more likely to abandon diets which demanded too strict a restriction of sugar and excluded all sweet foods.

The total amount of fat in your diet should provide no more than 33 per cent of your total calories each day.

- For a woman eating 1940 calories a day, this amounts to 71g fat per day.
- Of this fat intake, the amount of saturated fat should be no more than 10 per cent of total calories. For a woman eating 1940 calories a day this amounts to 21.5g of fat per day:
  $1940 \times 10\% = 194$ calories
  1g fat = 9 calories
  $194 \div 9 = 21.5$g fat

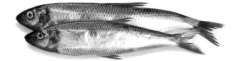

# Other Vital Nutrients

## Dietary Fibre

Although it passes though our digestive tract unchanged, fibre is essential for a healthy digestive system. Fibre consists of a number of compounds such as pectin, hemicellulose, lignin and gums, all of which are found in the cell walls of plants.

Broadly, there are two groups of fibre. Insoluble fibre is mainly in wheat, especially bran, and wholegrain cereals, fruit, vegetables and pulses. It absorbs water, making stools larger, softer and easier to pass. This helps prevent constipation and straining, which can help prevent haemorrhoids (piles) and diverticular disease – a condition where muscle spasms in the colon cause abdominal pain and disturbance to normal bowel function. It also speeds up the rate at which waste material is passed thorough the body. This is believed to play an important role in preventing bowel cancer.

Soluble fibre, in oats and oat bran, beans, pulses and some fruits, can lower high blood-cholesterol levels and slow the absorption of sugar into the blood stream.

The recommended intake of fibre for men and women is 18g per day, but surveys show that only one in ten of us eat this amount. Easy ways to increase your fibre intake include:

- Choose a wholegrain cereal that provides 3g of dietary fibre or more per serving, such as porridge, muesli or bran flakes at breakfast.
- Choose wholemeal or granary bread. Look for the words wholegrain, wholewheat and wholemeal on the label.
- Eat more beans and pulses by adding them to soups and casseroles.
- Eat a minimum of five servings of fruit and vegetable a day.
- Try ready to eat dried fruits as a snack or add them to your breakfast cereal.
- Use brown instead of white rice and choose wholemeal pasta.

## Salt (sodium chloride)

Sodium plays a vital role in the body's fluid balance as well as being involved in muscle and nerve activity. However, almost all of us consume far more than we actually need or is good for us. Eating too much salt is believed to be a major factor in the development of high blood pressure, which increases the risk of stroke and heart disease. High intakes can also cause leeching of calcium from the bones, increasing the risk of osteoporosis and may aggravate asthma, cause water retention and increase the risk of stomach cancer. Experts recommend reducing our salt intake to no more than 6g per day (equivalent to 2.4g sodium), which is around half most people's intake. About 80 per cent of the sodium in our diet comes from processed foods: one small tin of chicken soup can contain over half the recommended daily amount.

Our taste for sodium and salt is something that increases the more we eat. In the same way we can teach our taste buds to enjoy foods with less sugar we can train them to enjoy foods with less sodium. If you gradually reduce the amount of salt you eat your taste buds will adapt as the sodium receptors on the tongue become more sensitive to salt. This process takes two to three weeks. Try using other flavourings such as herbs and spices, lemon or mustard to flavour your foods. As a general rule, foods that contain more than 0.5g of sodium per serving are high in sodium. Foods that contain less than 0.1g of sodium per serving are low in sodium.

## Water

Water is vital to good health. The fact that we could survive for several weeks without food but only a few days without water demonstrates just how important it is. Depending on factors such as your age, sex and how much muscle you have, water accounts for 55–75 per cent of your total body weight – for an average adult that's between 45 and 54 litres! Water is essential to every organ, every cell and every tissue in the body: it helps regulate body temperature; transports nutrients and oxygen to cells; it is essential for the elimination of waste products; it is necessary to make saliva and digestive juices; it is essential for digestion and is used to lubricate joints. It also acts as a protective cushion for organs and tissues.

Unlike some other nutrients, the human body does not store water, so you need to provide a regular supply. The average adult loses about 2.25 litres of water every day through the normal functioning of the body. If the weather is hot, you are doing lots of exercise or you work in an air-conditioned office, you'll lose even more. Some foods – particularly fruit and vegetables – contain plenty of water. A slice of watermelon for example, is 92 per cent water while an apple is 84 per cent water. But while they can help replace some of the water lost each day, we still need to drink around 1.8 litres of fluid a day to prevent the body becoming dehydrated.

About 85 per cent of our brain tissue is water, which perhaps explains why even mild dehydration can lead to headaches, lethargy, dizziness and an inability to concentrate. Long-term dehydration can lead to digestive problems, kidney problems and joint pain. Relying on thirst to tell you when you need to take a drink is not advisable – by the time you feel thirsty, the body is probably already mildly dehydrated. Anything that contains caffeine, such as tea, coffee or cola drinks, as well as alcohol, will act as a diuretic, encouraging the body to excrete water. An easy way to check to see if you are drinking enough fluid is to take a look at your urine. If you are drinking enough it should be a light yellow colour; if it's dark yellow, that's a sign you're not drinking enough.

Aim to drink at least eight to ten glasses of fluid a day (in warm weather you'll need to drink more). Eating plenty of fruit and vegetables will help increase your fluid intake. Take water breaks rather than coffee breaks at regular intervals during the day – keeping a bottle of water on your desk at work will remind you to have a drink. Remember that it's essential to drink plenty of water before, during and after taking exercise, especially when the weather is warm.

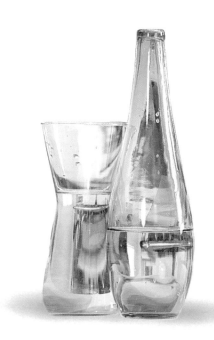

# 2

The Philosophy Behind
Body Control Pilates®

# The **Eight Principles**
## of Body Control Pilates®

There are eight principles behind the
Body Control Pilates Method

- relaxation

- concentration

- alignment

- breathing

- centring

- co-ordination

- flowing movements

- stamina

# Relaxation

There is a wonderful line in *The Bonesetter's Daughter* by Amy Tan when the main character, Ruth, talks about her preferred form of exercise, 'Stress – clench muscles, hold for twelve hours, release for a count of five, then clench again.'

Sound familiar? Most of us suffer from some form of stress. Next time you feel yourself under pressure, stop and take note which parts of your body are tense – jaw? neck? shoulders? back? – those tight knots the masseur's fingers so expertly probe, that sweet agony as the knots unwind.

It is often very hard for these muscles to release, it's easier for them to stay 'switched on'. Therefore, one of our first priorities is to help you learn how to switch them off – to make sure that everyday stress isn't brought into a session. But by relaxed we do not mean collapsed – we need you ready to exercise, to move freely using the right muscles to make the movements.

The Relaxation Position is a good way to start a session – you will also notice that we use it as the starting and finishing position for many of the exercises.

## The Relaxation Position

- Lie on your back with a small towel or a firm, flat cushion underneath your head, if necessary, to allow the back of the neck to lengthen.
- Keep your feet parallel and hip-distance apart, that is, in a line with the centre of your buttocks. Your knees are bent.
- Place your hands on your lower abdomen.

In this position you can easily run through a checklist. Ask yourself:

- Am I holding tension in my neck and shoulders? If so, allow your neck to soften and your shoulders to widen and melt into the mat.
- Does my low back feel tight? Check that you have kept the natural curves of your spine, see page 32, then allow the spine to lengthen. Imagine you have dry sand in your back pockets and allow it to trickle out gently.
- Is my pelvis in neutral? Is my sacrum square on the mat? The sacrum is a fused bone in the back situated between the hip bones. Go through the Compass exercise on page 39.
- Are my thighs tense? You may have to adjust where you place your feet, bringing them nearer to your bottom or taking them further away.
- Have I got my knees in a line with my hips? Try lining them up with the middle of each buttock cheek.
- Can I feel the three points on the soles of my feet in contact with the floor – base of the big toes, base of the small toes, centre of the heels? When you have completed your checklist, you can start any exercise confident your alignment is good and that you have let go of any unnecessary tension. However, you will need to remain vigilant when you perform an exercise or those overactive, dominant muscles will kick back in.

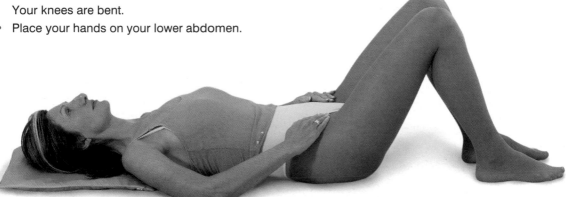

# Concentration

Hand in hand with relaxation is concentration. Pilates is a mental and physical conditioning programme that should train both mind and body. It requires you to focus on each movement made and develops your body's sensory feedback or proprioception, so that you know where you are in space and what you are doing with every part of your body for every second you are moving. Although the movements themselves may become automatic with time, you still have to concentrate because there is always a further level of awareness to reach. Use the exercises in this book to train your mind–body connection and you will find that you are far more body aware, not just when you exercise but in your daily activities as well. You will be able to concentrate better and will be far more co-ordinated in your movements. Learn to listen to the natural intelligence of your body – it really does talk to you!

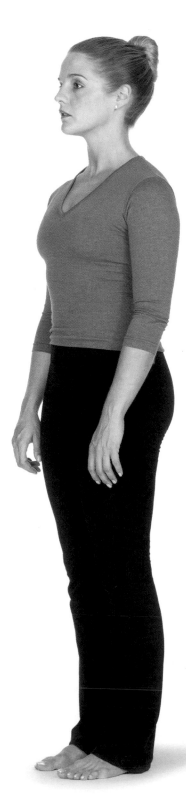

**Standing Correctly**

Imagine a balloon attached to the top of your head lifting you up through the spine.

Allow your neck to release.

Open your chest (without arching the back) by relaxing your shoulder blades down into your back.

Soften your armpits and direct your elbows away from your body.

Keep lifting up out of your hips.

Check that the pelvis is in neutral (page 39), that the pubic bone and the hip bones are in line and that the muscles at the front of the hips are soft.

Release your knees.

Are your feet hip-distance apart? Keep the weight evenly balanced on both feet – do not allow them to roll in or out. Remember the three points: base of the big toe, base of the small toe, centre of the heel.

# Alignment

By constantly reminding the body of how it should be standing, sitting or lying and by moving correctly, you can bring it into better alignment – essential not only to restore muscle balance but to look good as well. Slouching is extremely unattractive – it makes you look shorter, fatter, round shouldered and even makes your breasts look droopy. Not very inspiring! Furthermore, if you exercise without concern for the correct position of the joints, you risk stressing them, which can lead to extra wear and tear.

Muscles have an optimal length at which they function best – if you have poor postural alignment this length may have been altered, and the muscles can end up too long or too short, either way their ability to do their job properly is affected. By placing your bones in the right place before you start an exercise and being aware of where they are while you do the exercise, you stand a good chance of getting the right muscles working. This ensures good movement which means that your workout is going to be really effective. What we are aiming for is for you to be able to recognize and keep your joints in their 'neutral' positions (page 33), that is in the ideal position for good muscle balance and healthy ligaments. Gradually, your body will 'remember' the positions and you will find yourself sitting correctly and walking taller.

We already have a checklist for the Relaxation Position. This next checklist should help you align your body correctly while standing:

Now, bring your focus to the head balancing freely over the ribcage, which is floating over the hips and the hips are floating over the feet. You are at once grounded through the soles of your feet, yet lengthening up through your spine. Keep the three main body weights, head, ribcage and pelvis balanced over each other.

Good standing is a dynamic exercise, which works all the deep postural muscles of the body.

**Finding Your Neutral Spine and Pelvis**

Many of the exercises require you to have your spine and pelvis in their natural neutral positions. For the spine this means the position where it keeps its length and its natural 'S' shape. This is where there is least stress on the facet joints – the bony protuberances on the back of the vertebrae – the ligaments and the discs, and which allows the muscles to be at their optimal length and so function normally when we move. The Compass on page 39 is designed to help you find the correct neutral position of the pelvis and the spine. Once you are familiar with this in the Relaxation Position (page 31), you should practise finding neutral while standing, sitting, in four-point kneeling and lying on your side so that it becomes normal. If the muscles round the pelvis are very out of balance, you may find neutral difficult to maintain. When this is the case, consult your medical practitioner or your Pilates teacher, as it is often necessary to work in what is the best neutral you can achieve. You may need to use support such as towels or flat cushions. Usually after a few months, as the muscles begin to rebalance, neutral becomes more comfortable.

# Breathing

*'Indefatigably and conscientiously practise breathing until the art of correct breathing becomes habitual, automatic and subconscious, which accomplishment will result in the bloodstream receiving its full quota of oxygen and thus ward off undue fatigue.'* Joseph Pilates

Improving your breathing is probably the single most dramatic difference you can make to your overall health – but, breathing is the one thing we all take for granted. Few of us breathe efficiently and what a waste that is, because we miss out on all that wonderful oxygen which nourishes and replenishes every cell in the body and also has an important role to play in burning calories and shedding fat. We may go to great expense to buy the latest 'oxygen-rich' skin creams or, at an extreme, even spend time in oxygen tents. But the best results are to be had by simply learning to breathe more effectively, increasing the lung capacity and using the lower lobes of the lungs as well as the upper. By taking the time to master lateral or thoracic breathing, you can, ultimately improve your hair, skin, nails, bones and your overall wellbeing. What's more, once this breathing becomes automatic, once it becomes your natural, unconscious way of breathing you will reap the benefits every second of the day and night.

# Centring: Creating a 'Girdle of Strength'

Joseph Pilates had no formal medical training, but he discovered that if he hollowed his navel back towards his spine, his low back felt protected and thus he introduced the direction 'navel to spine' for all his exercises. He called the area between the hips and the ribcage 'the powerhouse' and taught that all movements should originate from this strong centre – this natural girdle of strength. In so doing, he was using his deep postural muscles to stabilize his spine – modern physiotherapists now call this core stability. The key muscles are transversus abdominis, the deepest of your abdominal muscles, and multifidus, a deep spinal muscle.

Think of the vertebrae of your spine being like a pile of books, stacked on top of each other. The role of transversus abdominis and multifidus is to stop one of the books slipping out of place; to prevent one vertebra from slipping too far off its neighbour, which can cause anything from facet-joint to disc problems. Unfortunately, poor posture, sitting for long periods of time and slouching often means that the deep stabilizing muscles are held lengthened and under stress. Add to this, having children, lack of exercise, or the wrong type of exercise, and it is easy to see why these deep postural muscles are weakened. The exercises on pages 41–3 will teach you how to locate and strengthen your deep stabilizing muscles.

Once you have learned to create a strong centre, we can start to challenge that stability by moving our limbs and adding movements such as rotation, flexion and extension. The exercises starting on page 44 will take you through this step by step.

## Co-ordination

So now you are relaxed, focused, aware and aligned. You are breathing efficiently (or learning to) and you have located and strengthened your deep core muscles. You are now ready to add movement. Step by step, the exercises will teach you how to move well. It may seem strange to begin with; it will feel different (after all, you have probably been moving badly for many years), but the movements soon become automatic or 'grooved' as they are locked into the body's memory. Meanwhile, the actual process of learning these new co-ordination skills is excellent mental and physical training, stimulating the two-way communication channel between mind and body.

## Flowing Movements

Pilates is all about natural movements performed smoothly, gracefully and with attention to detail. You will not be required to twist into awkward positions or to strain. We start with small movements and build up to more complicated combinations – the idea is for you to be constantly challenged. As beginners, you need to keep your limbs close to you, rather than risk losing your alignment and stability, but as you grow more confident and proficient you will be able to take your joints through their full range of motion.

   Whatever exercise you are performing, the movements must be precisely executed with control. The movements are generally slow, lengthening away from a strong centre, which gives you the opportunity to check alignment and focus on using the right muscles. Slow doesn't mean easy though – in fact it is harder to do an exercise slowly than quickly and it is also less easy to cheat!

## Stamina

Stamina is both a goal and an end result of Pilates. We wish to build strength, endurance and stamina into the body. We can do this by challenging stability, working with longer levers (for example an extended leg rather than a bent one), adding load with weights, using resistance or unstable surfaces. Many people complain of tiredness after a day on their feet, simply because standing badly is tiring: the ribcage is compressed and, as a consequence, the lungs are constricted. As you learn to open and lengthen the body, breathing becomes more efficient. All Pilates exercises are designed to encourage the respiratory, lymphatic and circulatory systems to function more effectively. As you become more proficient at the exercises and your muscles begin to strengthen and work correctly, you will discover that your overall stamina improves dramatically. You will no longer be wasting energy holding on to unnecessary tension or moving inefficiently. Your body will move as nature intended.

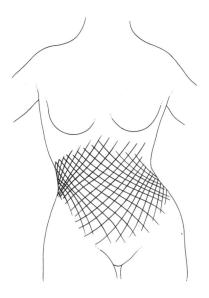

# 3

## The Exercise Programme

# Basics of Body Control Pilates®

We are now going to teach you the skills you need to perform the exercises well. Once you have mastered one skill you can move on to the next, layering one level on another. You will also find that learning one skill helps with the others. Remember how you felt on your first driving lesson? There was so much to remember – steering, clutch, gears, brake, mirrors, signals, etc. Then, all of a sudden, everything fell into place and you drove easily without having to think about it, even so, you still watch the road! It becomes simple because driving a car has entered your muscle memory banks, alongside learning how to swim, ride a bike and so on. It's exactly the same with Pilates. At first you may despair – keeping neutral, breathing wide, zipping up and hollowing – but, eventually, it all comes together and you can move on.

The basic skills you need to begin are breathing, good alignment and centring.

# Breathing

Stand in front of a mirror and watch as you take a deep breath. Do your shoulders rise up round your ears? Does your lower stomach expand when you breathe in? Most of us breathe inefficiently. Ideally, you should breathe wide and full into your back and sides. This makes sound sense because the lungs are situated in the ribcage and by expanding it, the volume of the cavity is increased and the capacity for oxygen intake is increased as well. It also encourages maximum use of the lower part of the lungs.

This type of breathing, thoracic or lateral breathing, makes the upper body more fluid and mobile. The lower ribcage expands wide as you breathe in and closes down as you breathe out. As you breathe in, your diaphragm automatically descends. The aim of thoracic breathing is not to stop this but to focus on the movement so it is widthways and into the back. The lungs need to expand in all directions as they fill with air. Unfortunately, for most of us, they never get to be fully inflated! Learning how to breathe thoracically will change that.

Joseph Pilates used to say, 'Squeeze out the lungs as you would wring a wet towel dry. Soon the entire body is charged with fresh oxygen from toes to fingertips.'

Try this simple exercise:
- Sit or stand tall. Bad posture compresses your ribcage.
- Wrap a scarf or towel round your ribs, crossing it over at the front.
- Holding the opposite ends of the scarf and gently pulling it tight, breathe in and allow your ribs to expand the towel (be careful you do not lift the breastbone too high).
- As you breathe out, gently squeeze the towel to help you fully empty your lungs. Relax the ribcage and allow the breastbone to soften.
- As you breathe out, you will also engage the pelvic floor muscles and hollow the abdomen (this is fully explained in Centring on page 40) which gives both lumbar and pelvic stability

as you move. Ultimately, you will need to keep these muscles engaged as you breathe in and out.

Also important to Pilates is the timing of the breath. Most people find this difficult at first, but once you have mastered it, it makes sense. As a general rule:
- You breathe in to prepare for a movement.
- You breathe out, zip up and hollow (page 41), and move.
- You breathe in, still zipped and hollowed, to recover.

Moving on the exhalation will enable you to relax into the movement and prevent you from tensing. It also offers greater core stability at the hardest part of the exercise and safeguards against holding the breath, which can unduly stress the heart and lead to serious complications.

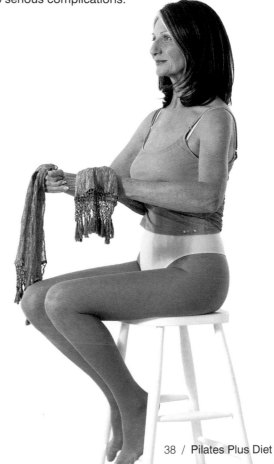

# Alignment

We have discussed at length the importance of good alignment (page 32).

Use the Relaxation Position on page 31 and Standing Correctly (page 32) to remind yourself how to position the body correctly. The following exercise will help you to find your neutral pelvis and spinal positions:

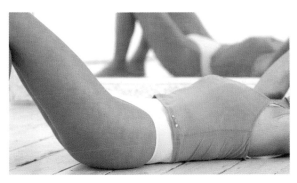

North

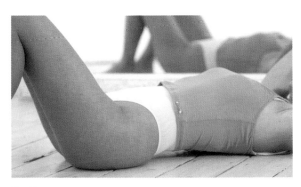

South

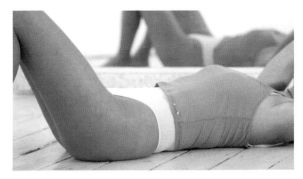

Neutral

**The Compass: Finding Neutral**

In Pilates, the aim is to work with the pelvis and spine in their natural, neutral positions. The angle of your pelvis affects the angle of your spine so learning how to find your neutral pelvis is the first step towards finding your neutral spinal position.

- Lie in the Relaxation Position. Checklist! (page 31).
- Imagine you have a compass on your lower abdomen. The navel is north and the pubic bone south, with west and east on either side. Now, we'll try two incorrect positions in order to help you find the correct one.
- Tilt your pelvis up towards north. The pelvis tucks under, the waist flattens and the curve of the low back is lost as your tailbone (coccyx) lifts off the mat. You will grip the muscles round your hips and abdominals.
- Next, carefully and gently move the pelvis in the other direction so that it tilts down towards south (avoid this bit if you have a back injury). The low back arches, the ribs flare and the stomach sticks out. Come back to the Relaxation Position.
- Aim for a neutral position between these two extremes. Go back to the image of the compass and think of the pointer as a spirit level. When you are in neutral, the pubic and pelvic bones will be level north/south and east/west. Your sacrum will rest squarely on the mat. You should feel as though the tailbone is lengthening away along the mat. Try to keep both sides of the waist long and equal.
- Now bring your awareness to your spine. Think of the 'S' shape of the spine (page 33). Think of lengthening through the spine while keeping those natural curves.

# Centring: The Pilates Powerhouse – Your Girdle of Strength

When Joseph Pilates taught his exercises, he used the direction 'navel to spine'. Eighty years on, we have adapted this instruction in the light of recent medical research which indicates that one of the best ways to activate the transversus abdominis muscle is to start the action from underneath – that is from the pelvic floor. Joseph Pilates was not wrong in teaching 'navel to spine' as this results in good stability – it is just that many people find engaging the pelvic floor muscles helps them to find transversus abdominis. This method gives the added bonus of developing good pelvic floor muscles which are essential for preventing incontinence, prolapses, prostate problems and, of course, enhancing your sex life.

One of the most important aspects in all stability work is engaging the muscles at the right amount of effort. Muscles can work from 0–100 per cent effort. Try standing up and tightening your buttocks as much as you can to 100 per cent. Now try to release them by about 50 per cent. Then let go half that again to 25 per cent – that's how much you should be working your deep muscles. This is because these muscles have to work for you all day every day. If you work them harder they will become fatigued, and they need endurance. For basic stability work we want you to work the muscles gently at no more than 25 per cent effort. Of course when you are doing an advanced exercise such as the Hundred on page 64, you will need to work a bit harder to stay stable. In these exercises it is important to engage transversus gently and slowly and then gradually increase the contraction.

Back to the pelvic floor. Where are your pelvic floor muscles? They are the muscles running from the front to the back of the body at the base of the abdomen, forming a hammock on which all your abdominal contents rest! For our exercises we need to isolate only parts of your pelvic floor muscles and to do so in a particular way. Be warned – this isn't easy and requires a lot of patience, a lot of practice and a lot of concentration!

We are trying to engage the muscles of the vagina for women and the urethra for both sexes (men should think about lifting their 'crown jewels'!). One way to help locate these muscles is to suck your thumb as you draw them up inside. It sounds crazy, but it is effective! You want to think about these muscles drawing together side to side and up a little. Think of how a camera shutter closes! At this stage we do not want you to engage the muscles around the anus, as it is too easy for the buttock muscles to kick in and substitute.

Try the Pelvic Elevator for awareness of where you are working and how hard you should work.

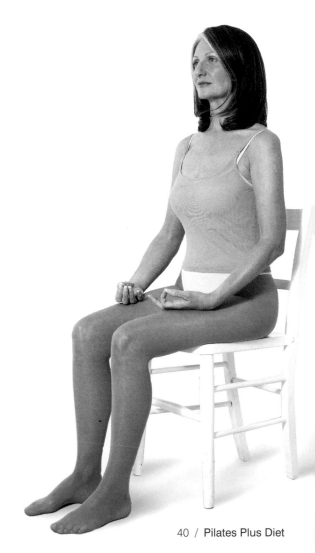

# The Pelvic Elevator  (*sitting*)

This exercise was created to isolate and engage the deep stabilizing muscles of the pelvis, pelvic floor and spine – transversus abdominis and multifidus. In order to achieve the best possible stability, you need to be able to contract the pelvic floor muscles at the same time as hollowing these lower abdominal muscles.

## Starting Position

Sit tall on an upright chair, making sure that you are sitting square, and with the weight even on both buttocks. Imagine your pelvic floor is like the lift in a building and this exercise requires you to take the lift up to different floors.

## Action

1  Breathe in wide and full into your back and sides, then lengthen up through the spine.
2  As you breathe out, draw up the muscles of your pelvic floor as if you are trying to stop the flow of urine. Remember to draw them together from side to side rather than front to back. Take the pelvic lift up to the first floor of the building. This is as far as you need to engage the muscles when given the instruction to zip up and hollow.
3  Breathe in and release the lift back to the ground floor.
4  It is useful to feel what it is like to pull the pelvic floor up further, so . . .
5  Breathe out and take the lift up to the second floor.
6  Breathe in and release.
7  Breathe out and take the lift up to the third floor.
8  Breathe in and relax.

## Watchpoints

• When you reached the first floor, you should have felt the deep lower abdominals engage. This is transversus abdominis coming into play. By starting the action from the pelvic floor, you encourage the 'six pack' muscle, rectus abdominis, to stay quiet. If you were to take the lift all the way to the top floor, you would probably be engaging the muscles at over 30 per cent and the six pack would take over – so keep the action low and gentle.
• Do not allow the buttock muscles to join in.
• Keep your jaw relaxed.
• Do not take your shoulders up to the top floor too – keep them down and relaxed.
• Try not to grip round your hips.
• Keep the pelvis and the spine quite still.

Once you have found your pelvic floor muscles it should be easier to isolate the transversus abdominis muscle. To engage this muscle correctly (at no more than 25 per cent) think of:

• hollowing
• scooping
• drawing back the abdominals towards the spine
• sucking in

The instructions for this action from now on will be 'zip up and hollow' – you need to imagine you are zipping up an internal zip from your pelvic floor upwards and, at the same time, hollowing the lower abdominals back to the spine. Remember, initially take the lift to the first floor only! Keep the action low and gentle.

The following two positions will help to ensure that this is done correctly.

# Stabilizing in Prone Lying

**Equipment**

A small, flat cushion.

**Starting Position**

Lie face down, resting your head on your folded hands. Open the shoulders out and relax the upper back (use the cushion under your abdomen if your low back is uncomfortable). Your legs are shoulder-distance apart and relaxed.

**Action**

1 Breathe in wide to prepare.
2 Breathe out and zip up and hollow.
3 Imagine there is a precious egg just above the pubic bone that must not be crushed. Do not tighten the buttocks – there should be no movement in the pelvis or the spine.
4 Breathe in and out, staying zipped, for a count of ten.
5 Repeat five times.

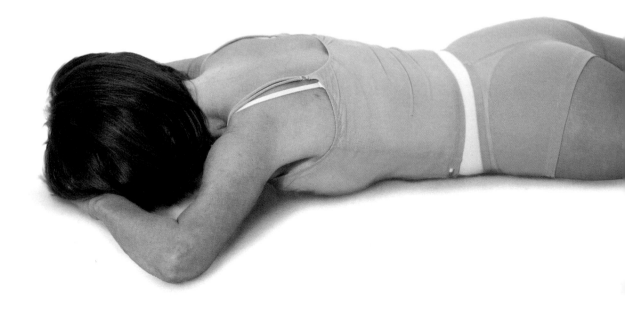

# Stabilizing in the Relaxation Position

**Starting Position**

Lie in the Relaxation Position (page 31) and go through the checklist. Find your hip bones (they are where hipster jeans would sit). Place your fingers an inch inwards and downwards from these bones and feel that the lower abdominals are relaxed.

**Action**

1 Breathe in wide to prepare and lengthen through the spine.
2 Breathe out and zip up and hollow – your fingers should feel your abdominals engage.
3 Breathe normally now, as you keep these muscles working – try to think of them sinking back towards the spine. If they bulk up or go very tight you are working too hard.
4 Work up to keeping zipped and hollowed for five breaths.

**Watchpoints**

- Check constantly that you are still breathing! And that your ribcage is moving!
- Do not allow the pelvis to tuck under – stay neutral with your pelvis level.
- Do not push into the spine. Keep your tailbone on the floor and lengthening away.

This, then, is your strong centre. For most of the exercises, you will be asked to zip up and hollow, engaging the pelvic floor muscles and drawing the lower abdominals back to the spine before and during your movements, lengthening away from a strong centre.

**Note:** remember that when doing the advanced exercises you should zip up and hollow gently, then slowly increase the hollowing action.

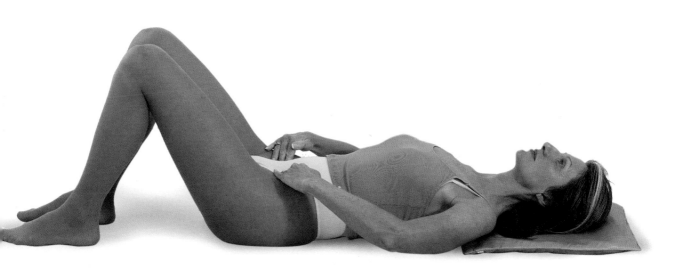

# Pelvic Stability – Leg Slides, Drops, Folds and Turnout

## Aim

Having mastered breathing, correct alignment and how to create a strong centre, learn how to add movement co-ordinating all this. It is not easy to begin with, but it soon becomes automatic. Meanwhile, the process of learning this co-ordination is fabulous mental and physical training as it stimulates that two-way communication between the brain and the muscles. Start with small movements, then build up to more complicated combinations.

Below are four movements to practise, all of them requiring you to keep the pelvis completely still. It is helpful to imagine that you have a set of car headlamps on your pelvis, shining up at the ceiling. The beam should be fixed, not mimicking searchlights! You can vary which exercises you practise each session but the starting position is the same for all four.

## Starting Position for Leg Slides, Drops, Folds and Turnout

- Adopt the Relaxation Position (page 31).
- Check that your pelvis is in neutral, your tailbone is down and lengthening away, then place your hands on your hip bones to check for unwanted movement.

## Action for Leg Slides

1 Breathe in wide and full to prepare.
2 Breathe out and zip up and hollow.
3 Sliding one leg away along the floor in line with your hips, keep the lower abdominals engaged and the pelvis still, stable and in neutral.
4 Breathe into your lower ribcage while you return the leg to the bent position, trying to keep the stomach hollow. Keep the foot in contact with the floor.
5 Repeat five times with each leg.

## Action for Knee Drops

1 Breathe in wide and full to prepare.
2 Breathe out and zip up and hollow. Allow one knee to open slowly to the side. Go only as far as the pelvis can stay still. It will want to roll from side to side – don't let it.
3 Breathe in still zipped and hollowed, as the knee returns to centre.
4 Repeat five times with each leg.

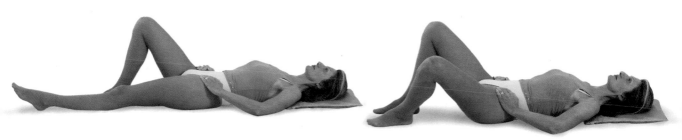

Leg Slides

Knee Drops

## Action for Knee Folds

With this movement it is particularly useful to feel that the muscles stay 'scooped' and do not bulge while you fold the knee in. Very gently, feel the muscles engage as you zip up and hollow.

1 Breathe in wide and full to prepare.
2 Breathe out and zip up and hollow. Fold the right knee up. Think of the thigh bone dropping down into the hip and anchoring there. If you find this very difficult you can bring your feet closer to you.
3 Do not lose your neutral pelvis – the tailbone stays down – and do not rely on the other leg to stabilize you. Imagine your foot is on a cream doughnut and you don't want to press down on it.
4 Breathe in and hold.
5 Breathe out and stay zipped and hollowed as you slowly return the foot to the floor.
6 Repeat five times with each leg.

**Warning for Turnout**: please take advice if you suffer from sciatica.

## Action for Turnout

This next action involves turning the leg out from the hip and is a preparation for exercises such as the Double Leg Stretch (page 68) where the legs are held in a turned-out position. It works the deep gluteal muscles, especially gluteus medius, which is one of the main stabilizing muscles of the pelvis.

1 Breathe in wide and full to prepare.
2 Breathe out and zip up and hollow. Fold the right knee up. Think of the thigh bone dropping down into the hip and anchoring there.
3 Breathe in.
4 Breathe out and remain zipped. Turn the right leg out from the hip bringing the right foot to touch the left knee if possible. Keep the knee in a line with the hip.
5 Do not allow the pelvis to tilt or twist or turn, keep it central and stable – headlamps to the ceiling!
6 Breathe in and then out, remaining zipped as you reverse the movement to return the foot to the floor.
7 Repeat five times to each side.

### Watchpoints for Leg Slides, Drops, Folds and Turnout

• Remember that you are trying to avoid even the slightest movement of the pelvis. It helps to think of the waist being long and even on both sides as you make the movements.
• Try to keep your neck and jaw released.

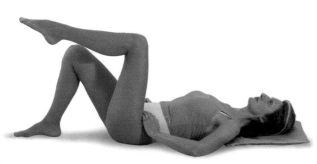

Knee Folds

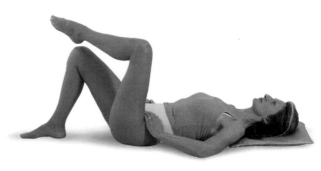

Turnout

# Scapular Stability

The final part of our girdle of strength concerns the muscles of the mid back, those which set the shoulder blades down. These are the lower trapezius and the serratus anterior muscles. If you are round shouldered, they are held lengthened and can weaken. When they are working correctly they stabilize the scapulae, placing them and the shoulder joint itself in the best position to allow for good movement. They also help to create a beautiful back and shoulders.

These exercises are designed to open out the chest, teach good alignment of the head, neck and shoulders and strengthen the stabilizing muscles. The idea is to re-educate your movements so that when you reach up with your arms the action is free flowing and natural.

To find these muscles, try this exercise:

**Back view:**

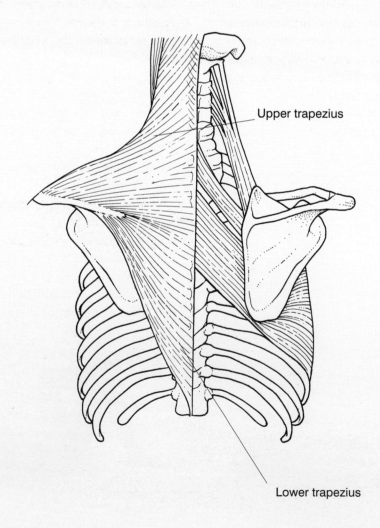

Upper trapezius

Lower trapezius

# Shoulder Reach

### Aim
To be aware of the muscles in the mid back, which connect the shoulder blades down into the back.

### Starting Position
Lie in the Relaxation Position (page 31). Have your arms resting down by your sides. Go through your Relaxation Position checklist.

### Action
1  Breathe in wide to prepare and lengthen up through the spine.
2  Breathe out and zip up and hollow. Slide your arms down towards your feet, reaching through your fingertips and turning your palms to face inwards. As you do so you will feel your shoulder blades connecting down into your back and your upper body opening out.
3  Breathe in and hold the stretch, be aware of the distance between your ears and your shoulders.
4  Breathe out and relax.
5  Repeat five times.

### Watchpoints
• There is a tendency for the ribcage to flare up as you slide the arms down. Keep the ribcage calm and down.
• Your neck should remain soft and released, the back of the neck stays long.

### Moving on
1  Follow directions 1–3 above then breathe out and, still reaching through your fingers, raise both arms until they are directly above your shoulders. As you do so, keep your upper shoulders soft and your elbows open.
2  Breathe in and lower.
3  Repeat five times.

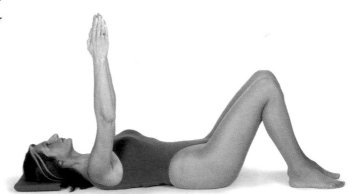

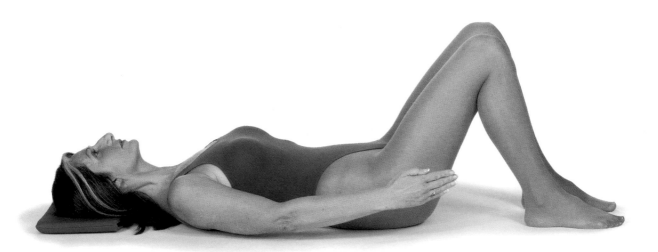

# The Dart *Stage One*

We are going to find the same muscles while lying face down.

## Equipment
A flat cushion (optional).

## Starting Position
Lie face down (you can place a flat cushion under your forehead to allow you to breathe) with your arms by your sides and your palms facing your body. Your neck is long, legs relaxed but parallel.

## Action
1 Breathe in to prepare and lengthen through the spine, tucking your chin in gently as if you were holding a ripe peach beneath it.
2 Breathe out and zip up and hollow. Slide your shoulder blades down into your back, lengthening your fingers down towards your feet.
3 The top of your head stays lengthening away from you too.
4 Keep looking straight down at the floor. Do not tip your head back.
5 Breathe in and feel the length of the body from the tips of your toes to the top of your head.
6 Breathe out, still zipping and hollowing, and release.

## Watchpoints
- Keep hollowing the lower abdominals.
- Do not strain the neck – it should feel released as your shoulders engage down into your back. Think of a swan's neck growing out between its wings.
- Keep your feet on the floor.
- Stop if you feel at all uncomfortable in the low back. This exercise can also be done with the feet hip-width apart and the thigh and buttock muscles relaxed.

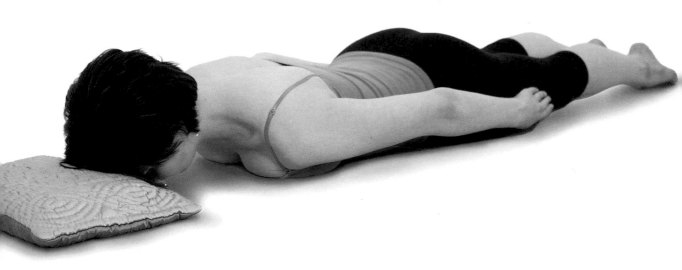

# Floating Arms

The muscles that you felt pulling your shoulder blades down into your back are the stabilizing muscles. Now that you have located them, try to feel them working in this exercise.

We all have a tendency to over-use the upper part of our shoulders (the upper trapezius). As you raise your arm, think of this order of movement:

- First, just your arm moves up and out.
- Then, you will feel the shoulder blade start to move – it coils down and round the back of the ribcage.
- Finally, the collarbone (clavicle) will rise up.

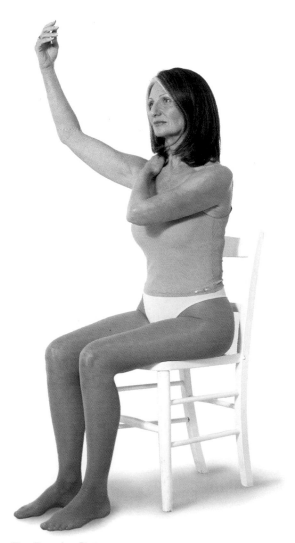

## Starting Position

Stand or sit tall. Put your left hand on your right shoulder so that you can feel your collarbone. You are going to try to keep the collarbone still for the first part of the movement, and your hand will check that the upper part of your shoulder remains 'quiet' for as long as possible. Very often this part over-works, so think of it staying soft and released, while the lower trapezius, the muscle below your shoulder blades, works to set the shoulder blades down into your back.

## Action

1. Breathe in to prepare and lengthen up through the spine, letting the neck relax.
2. Breathe out and zip up and hollow. Slowly begin to raise the arm, reaching wide out of the shoulder blades like a bird's wing. Think of the hand leading the arm and the arm following the hand as it floats upwards.
3. Rotate the arm so that the palm opens to the ceiling as the arm reaches shoulder level. Try to keep the shoulder under your hand as still as possible and the shoulder blades dropping down into your back as long as possible.
4. Breathe in as you lower the arm to your side.
5. Repeat three times with each arm.

## Watchpoints

- Keep a sense of openness in the upper body.
- Do not allow your upper body to shift to the side, keep centred.
- Let the hand lead the movement – reaching through the middle finger.

# The Starfish

## Aim

To combine everything you have learnt so far!
To have free-flowing movement away from a strong
centre. And, of course, don't forget your girdle
of strength.

## Stage One: The Upper Body

### Starting Position

Lie in the Relaxation Position (page 31) with your
arms down by your sides.

### Action

1  Breathe wide into your lower ribcage to prepare.
2  Breathe out and zip up and hollow. Move one
   arm in a backstroke movement as if to touch the
   floor above your head. Do not force the arm to
   touch the floor, move it only as far as is
   comfortable. Keep it soft and open, and the
   elbow bent. The shoulder blade sets down into
   your back. The ribs stay calm. Do not allow the
   back to arch at all.
3  Breathe in as you return the arm to your side.
4  Repeat five times with each arm.

## Stage Two: The Full Starfish

We are going to co-ordinate the opposite arm and
leg movement, away from our strong centre. This is
a sophisticated movement pattern, using all the
skills of good movement learnt so far.

### Starting Position

Lie in the Relaxation Position (page 31), with your
arms down by your sides.

### Action

1  Breathe in wide and full to prepare.
2  Breathe out and zip up and hollow.
3  Slide the right leg away in a line with your hips
   and take the left arm above you
   in a backstroke movement. Keep the pelvis
   neutral, stable and still and the stomach muscles
   engaged. Keep a sense of width and openness
   in the upper body and shoulders. Think of the
   shoulder blades setting down into your back.
4  Breathe in, still zipped and hollowed, and return
   to the Starting Position.
5  Repeat five times, alternating arms and legs.

### Watchpoints

- Do not be tempted to overreach – the girdle
  of strength must stay in place.
- Slide the leg in a line with the hip.
- Do not force the arm down to the floor.
- Ribs stay calm.

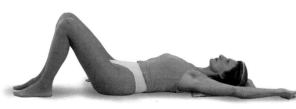

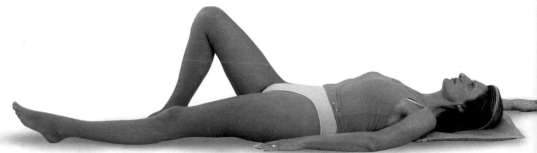

# The Exercises

In the following exercises you will be using all the basic skills from the last section. We suggest you read through all the exercises, taking time to study and practise each in turn, then you may start the workouts listed in chapter 6. We have given you different versions of some exercises and indicated their levels of difficulty: beginners, intermediate, advanced. Exercises without a grade are for all levels. Use your judgement as to when you have the strength and proficiency to move up a level.

# Spine Curls with Cushion

This wonderful exercise works on the mobility of the spine. Joseph Pilates always referred to using the spine 'like a wheel', encouraging his clients to peel their vertebra from the floor bone by bone. The good news is that it also works the buttocks and the inner thighs.

## Equipment
A plump cushion.

## Starting Position
Lie in the Relaxation Position (page 31), checking that your feet are parallel but a few centimetres apart and about 30 centimetres from your buttocks. Place the cushion between your knees. Your arms are relaxed down by your side, palms down.

When you are familiar with this exercise, you may try taking your arms above your head, shoulder-width apart, but only if, when you do this, your ribcage stays down – it should feel comfortable.

## Action
1 Breathe in wide to prepare.
2 Breathe out, zip up and hollow, and stay zipped throughout. Squeeze the cushion between the knees and curl the tailbone off the floor just a little.
3 Breathe in, and slowly curl back down to neutral, lengthening out the spine.
4 Breathe out, still zipped, and peel a little more of the spine off the floor.
5 Breathe in, and then breathe out, as you place the spine back down, bone by bone.
6 Continue to curl more of the spine off the floor each time you go up on the exhalation. Inhale while you are raised and exhale as you wheel the spine, vertebra by vertebra, back down on the floor. Aim to lengthen the spine as you wheel back down. Keep squeezing the cushion between the knees.
7 Do five full curls before you relax.

## Watchpoints
• You must not arch the back. Keep in your mind the image of a whippet who has just been scolded with his tail (your tailbone) curled between his legs!
• Keep the weight even on both feet and try not to let the feet roll in or out.
• Keep your neck long and soft.
• Do not come up any higher than your shoulder blades.

# Studio Adductor Stretch

A lovely exercise for helping you to still the mind and focus on your breathing, on the opening and lengthening of the spine, on the position of the shoulder blades and on the symmetry of the body.

## Equipment
A rolled-up towel (optional).

## Starting Position
Sit tall with your knees bent and the soles of your feet together. The feet should be a comfortable distance away. Check your pelvis is square and that you are sitting on your sitting bones. To find your sitting bones, sit on a chair and put your hands under your buttocks. If you wriggle around you will feel them – they are quite prominent. You may like to sit on a rolled-up towel which will help to position your pelvis and spine.

## Action
1 Breathe in wide to prepare and lengthen up through the spine.
2 Breathe out and zip up and hollow. Lift up out of your hips. Come forward as if coming up and over an imaginary beach ball. Your hands can cross and hold opposite ankles or rest softly on the floor in front of you.
3 Take twelve breaths in this position, breathing into your lower ribcage and back. Be aware of the bony bumps of the spine opening (imagine a dinosaur's back).
4 Tuck your chin in gently and check that you have lengthened up through the top of the head without hunching the shoulders, the shoulder blades should remain down into the back.
5 You may feel a gentle stretch in your inner thighs.
6 After twelve breaths, slowly unfurl on an out breath, zipping up and rebuilding the spine vertebra by vertebra until, finally, the head comes up.

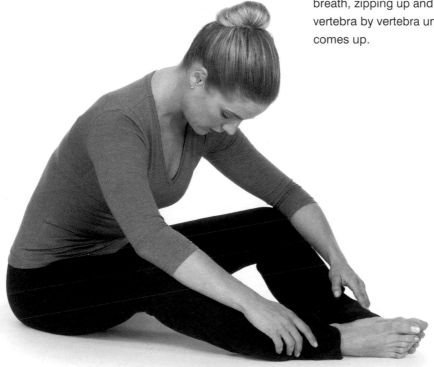

# Beach Ball Hamstring Stretch

Another great exercise to prepare the body for a workout as it helps you to focus on your body. Please take advice if you have a knee injury.

## Equipment
A rolled-up towel (optional).

## Starting Position
Straighten one leg out in front of you, in a line with your hip and with the knee cap facing the ceiling. The sole of the foot of your bent leg is resting on the inside of your other knee. Your foot is relaxed. If you find it easier you may like to sit on a rolled-up towel.

## Action
1  Breathe in to prepare and lengthen up through the spine.
2  Breathe out and zip up and hollow. Lift up out of your hips and gently stretch forward. Do not twist over one leg but stay in the centre.
3  Take twelve breaths in this position, breathing wide and full into the lower ribcage and back and relaxing into the stretch. Your neck is long, your chin is tucked in gently, your shoulder blades are down into your back.

4  Rest the same arm as the straight leg by the side of that leg. The arm on the bent-leg side goes behind you, palm facing up – this helps to keep the body square.
5  Make sure that both sides of your waist stay equally long. Once again, focus on the spine opening and lengthening.
6  After twelve breaths, on an out breath, zip up and hollow, and slowly rebuild the spine vertebra by vertebra.
7  Repeat on the other side.

## Watchpoints
* Keep the top of your head lengthening away, your jaw relaxed and your chin gently tucked in.
* Keep the weight even on both sitting bones.
* Do not lock the knee back, the straight leg stays straight but relaxed.

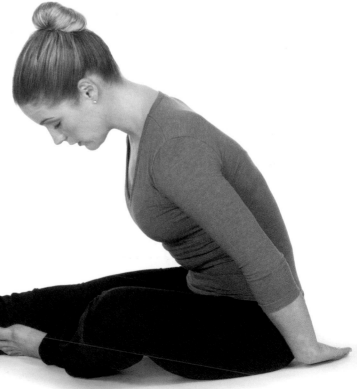

# Windows

## Aim

A lovely exercise to open the upper body and teach good mechanics. It also promotes flexibility and mobility round the shoulder joint.

Take advice if you have a shoulder injury.

## Equipment

A broomstick or a scarf (optional).

## Starting Position

Lie in the Relaxation Position (page 31). Raise your arms directly above your shoulders, palms facing forwards. If you are using a stick or a scarf, hold it gently and have your hands wide apart.

## Action

1 Breathe in wide and full to prepare.
2 Breathe out, zip up and hollow, and stay zipped throughout. Bring your elbows down towards the floor, so that your upper arms are on the floor in a line with the shoulders to each side, but your forearms still point towards the ceiling.
3 Breathe in and very slowly rotate your arms backwards so that the back of your hands come down towards the floor. Under no circumstances force the arms back, stop where they are comfortable. Feel your shoulder blades connecting down into your back as you make this movement.
4 Breathe out as you slowly straighten the arms along the floor (or just off the floor if this is more comfortable) keeping them wide. Don't lock the elbows. Keep the action smooth and flowing, but don't forget the shoulder-blade connection down in your back.
5 Breathe in as you raise the arms back to the Starting Position.
6 Repeat eight times.

## Watchpoints

* Make sure your movements are smooth and controlled and without strain.
* Ribcage down at all times.
* Do not force the arms down to the floor.

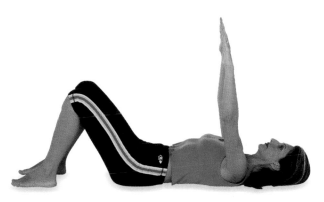

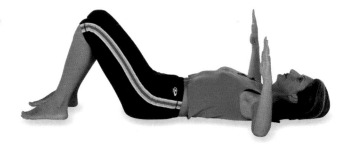

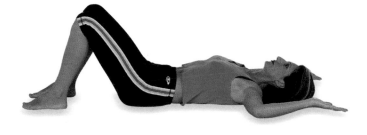

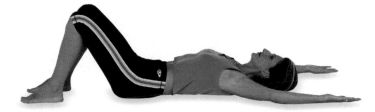

# Single Leg Circles

A classical Pilates exercise that tones the thighs, buttocks and the muscles round the hips. It also mobilizes the hips. You need to use your deep girdle of strength to steady your torso so this is an abdominal exercise as well!

**Starting Position**

Lie in the Relaxation Position (page 31). You will need to stay aware throughout the exercise of what is happening to your torso while the leg moves.

**Action**

1  Breathe in wide to prepare and lengthen through the spine.
2  Breathe out, zip up and hollow and stay zipped throughout. Bend your right leg in towards your chest. If you wish you may straighten the other leg along the floor (fig. 2) as it can remain bent for extra stability (fig. 1).

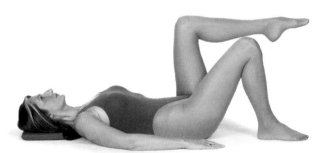

Fig. 1

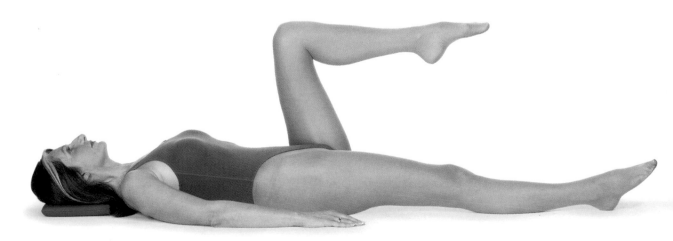

Fig. 2: Beginners (you may straighten one leg along the floor if you wish)

**3** You are now going to circle the leg from the hip joint, first moving it across the body then taking it outwards and back to the starting position. Keep the circles small to start with. The idea is that the pelvis and the rest of your body stay still and anchored. You are going to breathe in as you circle in and across the body, out as the leg moves away and back. Use your full girdle of strength to keep the body anchored and still, this means staying zipped and setting the shoulder blades down into the back, you may press your shoulder blades into the floor. Your arms will naturally help you to stay stable, but do not rely on them to keep you still – use your core strength.

**4** Repeat five circles each way with each leg.

**Watchpoints**

- Move the leg from the hip joint itself.
- The pelvis stays still and neutral.
- Keep checking that there is no unnecessary tension in the upper body.
- If your leg is straight, try not to lock out the knee.

**Moving On**

For intermediate level have both legs are straight: one along the floor and the other extended into the air. For advanced level have both legs straight and make bigger circles. Focus on the upswing of the circle.

How far you can straighten your leg will depend on the flexibility of your hamstrings. Although we are aiming for the leg to be straight, it is perfectly acceptable for it to remain slightly bent.

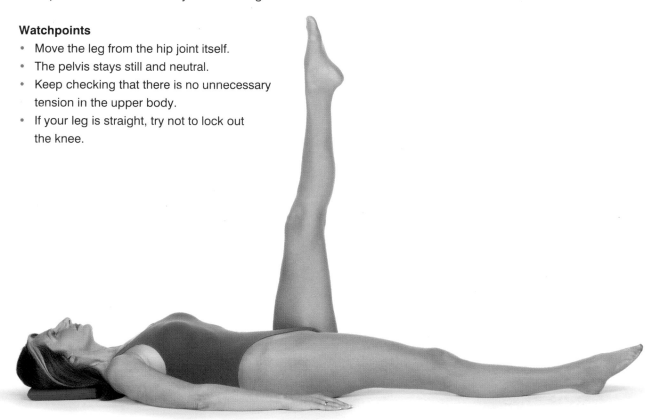

Intermediate (Advanced make wider circles)

# Curl Ups

Just look at the number of Watchpoints for this exercise, which you can see being done in any gym in the country. The reason our version works so well is that you are required to pay close attention to maintaining neutral and keeping your lower abdominals hollow. This ensures that transversus abdominis stays engaged and that you are targeting the right abdominal muscles to achieve the ultimate flat stomach. If you lose neutral, let your abdominals bulge or fling yourself up quickly, you lose the effectiveness of the exercise and that flat stomach will remain a dream!

## Starting Position

Lie in the Relaxation Position (page 31). Gently release your neck by rolling the head slowly from side to side. Lightly clasp your hands behind your head to cradle and support it (at no point should you pull on your neck). Keep your elbows open just in front of your ears throughout.

## Action

1 Breathe in wide and full to prepare.
2 Breathe out, zip up and hollow and stay zipped. Soften your breastbone, tuck your chin in a little (as if holding a ripe peach) and curl up, breaking from the breastbone. Your stomach must not pop up. Keep the pelvis level and the tailbone down on the floor lengthening away.
3 Breathe in and slowly curl back down, controlling the movement.
4 Repeat ten times.

**Warning:** avoid this exercise if you have neck problems.

## Watchpoints

- Try not to grip round the hips, keep those muscles soft.
- Stay in neutral, tailbone down on the floor and lengthening away. The front of the body keeps its length. A useful image is that there is a strip of sticky tape along the front of the body which should not wrinkle!
- Think of peeling the upper spine, bone by bone, from the floor.
- Think of the ribs funnelling down towards the waist.
- Keep the chin gently tucked in. Keep your neck released.
- Do not close your elbows as you come up – keep them open but within your peripheral vision.

## Moving on

Take an extra breath while curled up and come back down on the out breath.

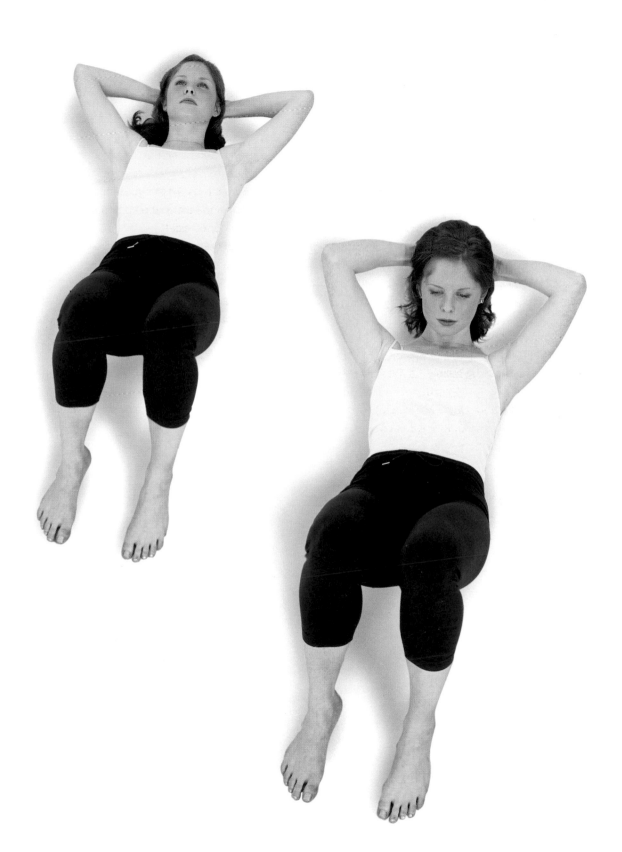

# Curl Ups with Leg Extension  (*intermediate*)

The additional challenge of extending your leg while curling up really helps to target the lower abdominals. Follow the directions very carefully to see dramatic results.

### Starting Position

Lie in the Relaxation Position (page 31) but have your feet closer together than normal, still lined up with (and parallel to) each other. Gently release the neck by rolling the head slowly from side to side. Clasp both hands lightly behind your head as for Curl Ups (page 58). Gently tuck in your chin as if holding but not squashing a large ripe peach.

**Warning:** avoid this exercise if you have neck problems.

### Action

1  Breathe in wide and full to prepare
2  Breathe out and zip up and hollow. Soften your breastbone and, breaking from the breastbone, curl up, making sure you stay in neutral. As you curl up, slowly extend your right leg, keeping the knee in line with your left knee. Your stomach must not pop up. Keep the length and width in the front of the pelvis and the tailbone down on the floor lengthening away. Do not tuck the pelvis or pull on the neck!
3  Breathe in, still zipped, and hold the position.
4  Breathe out and slowly curl back down, bending the knee back down at the same time.
5  Repeat five times with each leg.

### Watchpoints

* As for Curl Ups on page 58.

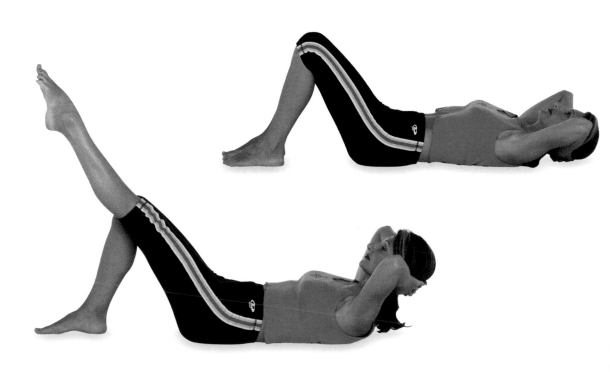

# Oblique Curl Ups

A great exercise for rediscovering your waistline, as it works the obliques, which wrap round your middle.

## Starting Position

Lie in the Relaxation Position (page 31). Clasp your hands lightly behind your head as for Curl Ups (page 58). Tuck your chin in – remember the ripe peach.

## Action

1   Breathe in wide and full to prepare.
2   Breathe out and zip up and hollow. Curl your upper body up and bring your left shoulder across towards your right knee. The right elbow stays back. Your stomach must stay hollow, the pelvis still, square and stable.
3   Breathe in, still zipped, and slowly lower with control.
4   Repeat five times to each side

## Watchpoints

*   The same Watchpoints as for Curl Ups apply (page 58).
*   Keep your sides equally long. There is always a tendency with this exercise to shorten one side of the waist as you come up. Keep the action simple, you are going across at an oblique angle.
*   Keep the upper body open, elbows back but in view.
*   Focus on keeping the pelvis very still, you may find that the opposite hip wants to come up, stay square and neutral.

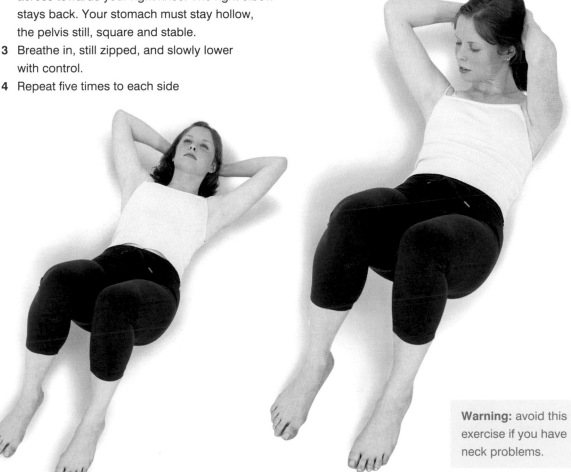

**Warning:** avoid this exercise if you have neck problems.

# The Double Knee Fold

## *Level One* (*beginners*)

This exercise looks deceptively easy, but is in fact one of the hardest exercises in the book. Bringing the knees up to the chest one at a time without allowing the lower abdominals to bulge and without losing neutral, requires excellent core stability. This Double Knee Fold is a part of the preparation for many classical exercises such as the Double Leg Stretch (page 68) or the Hundred (page 64).

We have given you two levels of difficulty. It is easier to learn Double Knee Folds in reverse – that is lowering the feet to the floor rather than lifting them off. Level One gives you some idea of the strength and control you will need to do Level Two.

**Starting Position**
Lie in the Relaxation Position (page 31).

**Action**
1 Breathe in wide and full to prepare.
2 Breathe out, zip up and hollow, and stay zipped throughout. Fold one knee up, staying in neutral and keeping the lower abdominals hollow as you did for Knee Folds (page 45).
3 Breathe in and lightly take hold of the raised knee, with one or both hands.
4 Breathe out and fold the second knee up so that both knees are now bent at an angle and it looks as though you are sitting on a chair (lying on your back of course). Line your feet up with the toes lightly touching. The knees stay hip-width apart.
5 Now for the hard bit. Let go of the knee, breathe in and lengthen through the spine, checking that your pelvis is in neutral and your low back feels anchored (using your zip).
6 Breathe out, still zipped, and slowly lower one foot to the floor – do not allow the abdominals to bulge or lose neutral.
7 Breathe in, then out and slowly lower the other foot.
8 Repeat six times, alternating which leg you raise and lower first.

**Watchpoints**
• You will be surprised at how the body tries to cheat and use everything other than the lower abdominals to stabilize you – be aware of this and keep your neck and shoulders relaxed.

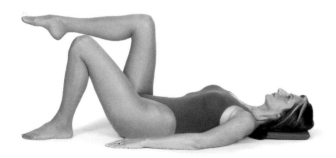

When you are happy you can do this version easily, you may raise and lower each leg, still one at a time, but on a single out breath. Then you can try Level Two.

# Level Two  (*intermediate*)

The Double Knee Fold is the starting position
for many of the classical exercises.

**Starting Position**
Lie in the Relaxation Position (page 31).

**Action**
1  Breathe in wide and full to prepare.
2  Breathe out, zip up and hollow and stay zipped
   throughout. Fold one knee up. The lower
   abdominals stay hollow and the pelvis neutral.
3  Breathe in wide and full.
4  Breathe out and fold the other knee up.
   Stay zipped, hollowed and neutral.
5  Breathe in wide.
6  Breathe out and lower the first leg you raised.
7  Breathe in, then out and lower the second leg.
8  Repeat six times, alternating which leg you
   raise and lower first.

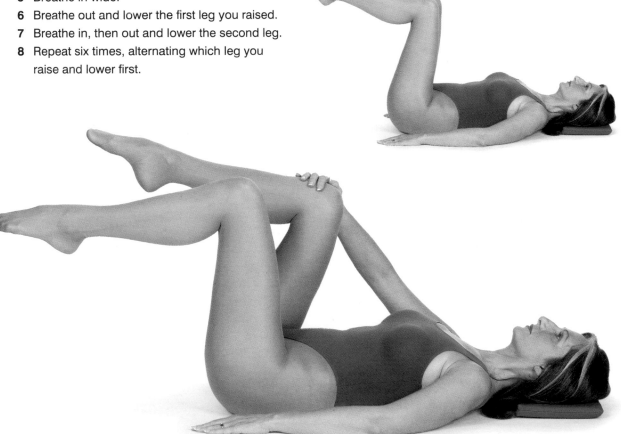

# The Hundred

**Aim**

To learn the breathing pattern of the Hundred, which involves lateral, lower ribcage breathing to a set rhythm. To strengthen the pectoral muscles. To master stabilizing the shoulder blades. To strengthen the abdominals. To energize the body.

The Hundred is one of the classical Pilates exercises. It used to be the warm-up exercise for mat classes. Well, it certainly warms you up! We have broken the exercise down into manageable, bite-sized chunks. When you have mastered one stage, you may proceed to the next. This unique exercise improves the efficiency of your respiratory system, stimulates the circulatory system, oxygenates the blood and boosts the lymphatic system as well as toning you from top to toe.

Please take advice if you have neck, back, respiratory or heart problems.

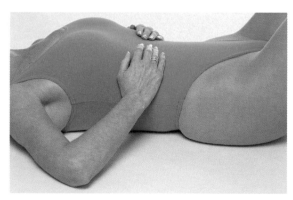

Stage One

**Stage One: Breathing Preparation (Beginners)**

• Lie in the Relaxation Position (page 31).

• Place your hands on your lower ribcage. Breathe in wide and full into your sides and back for a count of five. Breathe out and zip up and hollow for a count of five.

• Repeat ten times, trying to stay zipped and hollowed for both the in and the out breaths. If you find a count of five too difficult try a count of three.

**Stage Two: Breathing, plus Pumping Arms (Intermediate)**

• Lie in the Relaxation Position (page 31).

• Your arms are extended alongside your body, palms down, wrists straight, connect your shoulder blades down into your back as for the Shoulder Reach (page 47).

• Your head remains down on the floor.

**Action**

1  Zipping and hollowing throughout, and breathing in wide into your sides and back, pump your arms up and down no more than fifteen centimetres off the floor for a count of five. The shoulder blades stay down with the fingers lengthening away.

2  Breathe out and pump the arms for a count of five.

3  Repeat ten times, then slowly Double Knee Fold down (page 62).

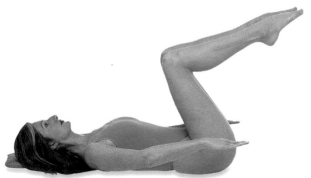

Stage Two

## Stage Three (Intermediate)
### Starting Position
Lie in the Relaxation Position (page 31).
Double Knee Fold (page 62) into the chair position, toes connecting, knees hip-width apart and parallel. Your arms are down by your sides. Slowly roll your head from side to side to release your neck.

### Action
1 Breathe in wide and full to prepare.
2 Breathe out and zip up and hollow. Curl the upper body off the floor remembering everything you learnt for Curl Ups (page 58): chin gently tucked forward, relaxed jaw, soft breastbone, released neck.
3 Still zipped and hollowed, start the breathing and the arm pumping action, which you mastered in the last exercise. Breathe in wide for five beats and out for five beats. Keep the shoulder blades down, fingertips lengthening away.
4 Repeat twenty times until you reach one hundred, then slowly Double Knee Fold down (page 62) and lower your head.

### Watchpoints
• Return to the floor if you feel any strain at all in your neck.
• To prevent strain and to engage the deep stabilizers, have your chin gently tucked in but not squashed. Your line of focus should be between your thighs. The back of your neck remains long, the front relaxed.
• You must keep breathing wide into your lower ribcage or you will become breathless. If you do feel breathless, stop at once.
• Keep a sense of width in your upper body. Do not close the shoulders in, keep the upper body open, the breastbone soft.
• Keep your back anchored to the mat.

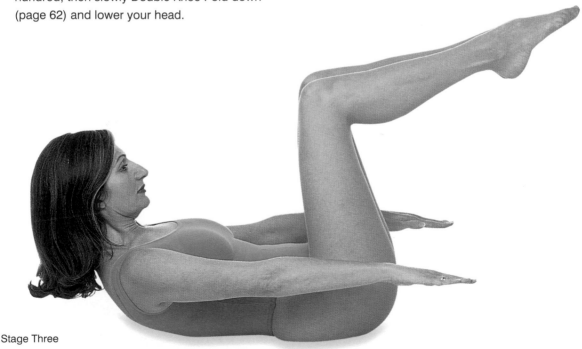

Stage Three

**Stage Four (advanced)**

**Starting Position**

Lie in the Relaxation Position (page 31). Double Knee Fold (page 62) into the chair position, toes connecting, knees hip-width apart and parallel. Your arms are down by your side. Slowly roll your head from side to side to release your neck.

**Action**

1 Breathe in wide and full to prepare.
2 Breathe out and zip up and hollow. Curl the upper body off the floor, remembering everything you learnt for Curl Ups (page 58): chin gently tucked forward, relaxed jaw, soft breastbone, released neck.
3 Breathe in and then out as, zipped and hollowed, you straighten the legs into the air as high as is comfortable. If this is difficult you can keep them bent. Do not allow them to fall away from you as this may cause your back to arch. Your back must stay anchored to the mat. Have your feet softly pointed.
4 Zipped and hollowed, start the breathing and pumping action of the arms, which you mastered in the last exercise. Breathe in wide for five beats and out for five beats. Keep the shoulder blades down, fingertips lengthening away.
5 Repeat twenty times until you reach one hundred, then slowly bend your knees down to your chest and lower your head.
6 Follow the instructions for Double Knee Fold (page 62) to get your feet on the floor.

**Watchpoints**

• Return to the floor if you feel any strain in your neck.
• To prevent strain and to engage the deep stabilizers, have your chin gently tucked in but not squashed. Your line of focus should be between your thighs. The back of your neck remains long, the front relaxed.
• You must keep breathing wide into your lower ribcage or you will become breathless. If you do feel breathless, stop at once.
• Keep a sense of width in your upper body. Do not close the shoulders in, keep the upper body open, the breastbone soft.
• Stay anchored. You will need to use your core muscles strongly.

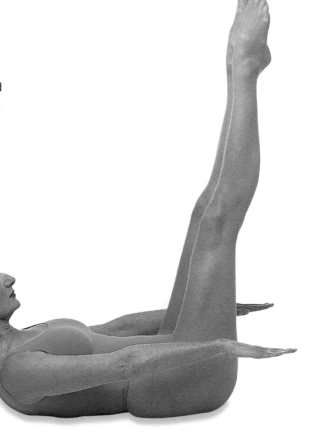

Stage Four

# The Full Hundred

**Stage Five (advanced)**

Stage Five is the same as Stage Four, except that this time when the legs are extended you turn them both out from the hip joints, and flex the feet towards you. Only do this if you have good hamstring length and can straighten your legs easily. The lower the angle of the legs the harder the abdominals will have to work to prevent your back from arching. Only lower them to 45° if you have excellent core stability.

# Double Leg Stretch

## Version One  (*intermediate*)

We have given you three versions of this classical abdominal exercise, for which you will need good core stability and co-ordination. It is Pilates at its finest!

### Starting Position
Lie in the Relaxation Position (page 31).
Double Knee Fold into the chair position (page 62): toes touching, knees hip-width apart and parallel. Clasp your hands lightly behind your head, keeping the elbows wide open. You should still be able to see them. Tuck your chin in gently.

### Action
1  Breathe in wide and full to prepare.
2  Breathe out, zip up and hollow, and stay zipped throughout. Slowly curl the head up from the floor, breaking from the breastbone and keeping the neck soft and long. As you do this, straighten the legs as much as is comfortable. Softly point the toes and keep your back anchored into the floor.
3  Breathe in, and slowly lower your head to the floor, bending the knees down to your chest.

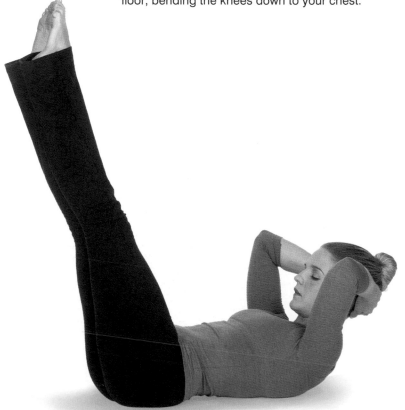

# Version Two  (advanced)

This is the Pilates Method at its very best –
a complex, choreographed sequence of movements
which effectively conditions the entire body, using
mind and body skills and free-flowing movements
round a strong centre.

**Starting Position**

Lie in the Relaxation Position (page 31). Double
Knee Fold into the chair position (page 62). Turn the
legs out from the hip socket, so that the knees open
from the hip – the toes are just touching but the
heels are apart. The lower legs are parallel to the
floor. Rest your hands on the outside of your knees,
keeping the elbows open. The breastbone is soft
and the shoulder blades are down into your back.
Gently roll your head from side to side to release
the neck.

**Warning:** avoid these exercises if
you have any neck or back injuries.

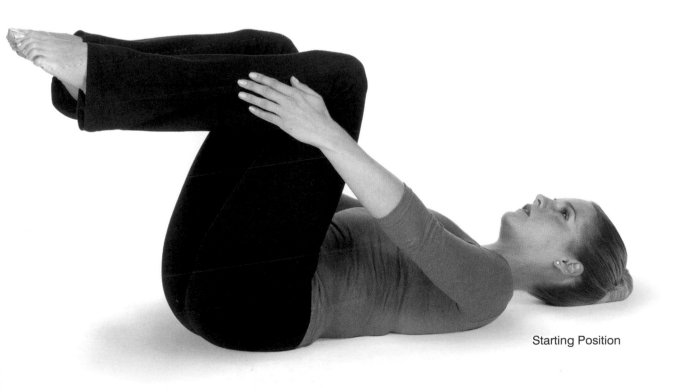

Starting Position

### Action

1  Breathe out and zip up and hollow. These core muscles should stay engaged throughout the exercise.

2  Breathe in and slowly curl your upper body from the floor, gently tucking in the chin. At the same time, straighten your legs into the air and turn them out from the hips. Flex the feet. Lengthen up from the inside of your legs to the heels. Squeeze the inner thighs together. Your arms are lengthening away from you at hip height.

3  Breathe out. Take your arms in a wide sweep up to the level of your ears (not behind) keeping the natural curve of the arms.

4  Breathe in as the arms circle down, round and come alongside the thighs.

5  Breathe out as you slowly lower your head back down on to the floor, bending the knees so that they are back in the Starting Position.

6  Repeat ten times.

### Watchpoints

- Do not allow the abdominals to bulge at all during the exercise – keep hollowing and keep lifting from the pelvic floor.
- Your eye line should be just above your knees, so that the chin stays tucked in and the back of the neck is long.
- With the legs turned out and straight, make sure that you anchor the head of your thigh bones into the hips.
- Do not allow the legs to fall away below an angle of 60° as this may cause your back to arch.
- Do not take your arms behind the level of your ears.
- Use your core muscles strongly.

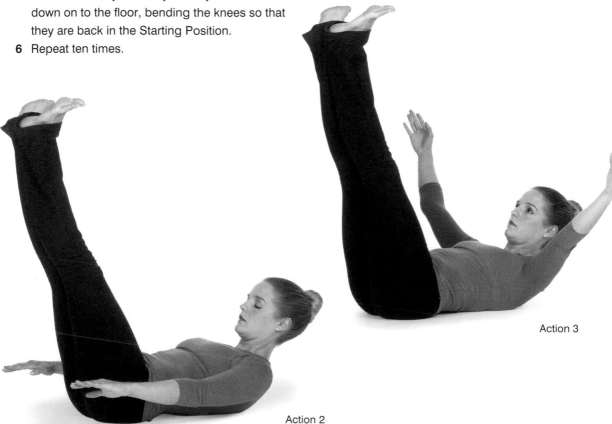

Action 2

Action 3

# Version Three (advanced)

This is a fun variation on the classical exercise, which requires you to get your timing just right.

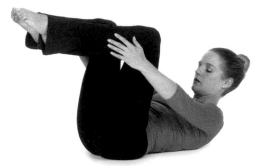

Starting Position

## Starting Position

Lie in the Relaxation Position (page 31). Double Knee Fold into the chair position (page 62): toes connected, knees hip-width in parallel, the lower legs are parallel to the floor. On the out breath zip up and hollow, curl the upper body from the floor and lightly clasp the outside of each knee or calf (wherever you can reach comfortably).

## Action

1 Breathe in wide and full to prepare, and stay zipped throughout. Straighten the legs into the air to about 70°; have your toes softly pointed. Simultaneously take the arms up directly behind you so that your body now forms a V shape. The palms face forwards; the arms are in a line with your ears. Reach through your fingers and toes and stay anchored.

2 Breathe out, bend the knees and sweep the arms back round in a large circle to clasp the outside of the knees.

3 Repeat five times, remaining curled up throughout.

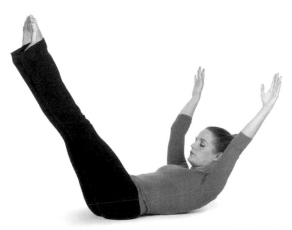

Action 1

## Watchpoints

• Do not lower the legs past 45° until you have very strong abdominals and excellent control.
• Feel that you are reaching through your fingertips away from your centre and that your toes are also reaching away from your centre.
• Do not overreach through the fingers. The arms stay in a line with the ears and the shoulder blades stay connected down into the back.
• Do not let your head fall back.

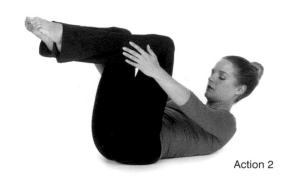

Action 2

# The Diamond Press

A subtle exercise, which has dramatic results. It really does help to reverse the effects of being hunched over all day. You can feel the tension in your neck release as the mid-back muscles, which stabilize the shoulder blades, slide them down into the back.

**Starting Position**

Lie on your front with your feet hip-width apart and parallel. Create a diamond shape with your arms by placing your fingertips together just above your forehead. Your elbows are open, your shoulder blades relaxed.

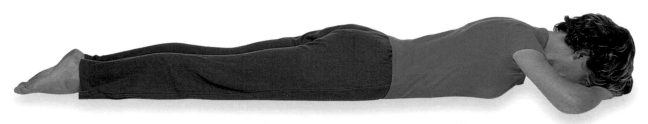

Starting Position

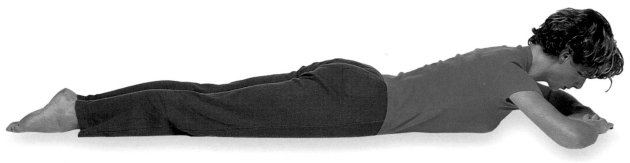

 Actions 2–3

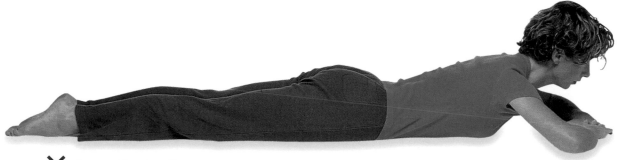

 Incorrect head position

## Action

1 Breathe in and lengthen up through the spine.

2 Breathe out, zip up and hollow, and stay zipped throughout. Slide the shoulder blades down into the back of your waist, simultaneously tucking your chin in (as if to hold the ripe peach), and extending your upper body three or four centimetres up off the floor. Stay looking down at the floor, the back of the neck is long – imagine a cord pulling you from the top of your head. Really make the connection down into the small of your back – you have to push a little on the elbows to come up, but this isn't a push-up so make the back muscles work.

3 Breathe in and hold the position. Keep the lower stomach lifted. The ribs stay on the floor.

4 Breathe out and slowly lower back down. Keep lengthening through the spine.

5 Repeat five times.

## Watchpoints

- Keep the lower abdominals drawing back to the spine.
- Make sure you keep looking down at the floor – if you lift your head back you will shorten the back of your neck.
- Really enjoy the sense of your neck growing out from between the shoulder blades.

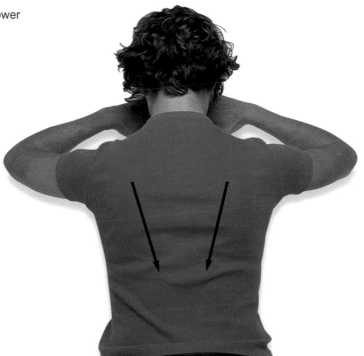

# The Dart *Stage Two*

The Dart strengthens the back muscles and helps to balance the body after the flexion involved with the abdominal curl ups. It also creates awareness of the shoulder blades and strengthens the muscles which stabilize them. This is a very important exercise in your programme.

**Equipment**
A flat cushion (optional).

**Starting Position**
Lie on your front. You may place a flat cushion under your forehead to allow you to breathe. Your arms are down at your sides, your palms facing your body. Your neck is long. Your legs are together, parallel and with your toes pointing.

**Action**
1 Breathe in to prepare and lengthen through the spine. Tuck your chin in gently
2 Breathe out, zip up and hollow, and stay zipped throughout. Slide your shoulder blades down into your back, and lengthen your fingers away from you down towards your feet. The top of your head stays lengthening away from your tailbone. Keep looking straight down at the floor. Do not tip your head back.

3 At the same time, squeeze your inner thighs together, but keep your feet on the floor, and slowly lift your upper body from the floor. Don't come up too high, just a few centimetres. Use your back muscles.
4 Breathe in and feel the length of the body from the tips of your toes to the top of your head.
5 Breathe out, still zipping, and lengthen and lower back down.
6 Repeat six times.

**Watchpoints**
- Keep hollowing the lower abdominals.
- Do not strain the neck, it should feel released as your shoulders engage down into your back. Think of a swan's neck growing out between its wings.
- Remember to keep your feet on the floor.

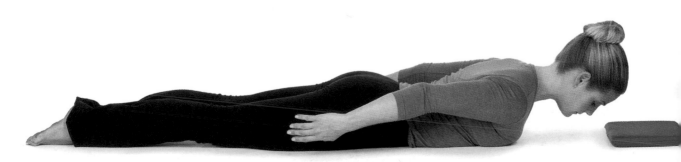

# The Star

This exercise works both the upper and lower body. It's great for toning the buttocks.

If you are uncomfortable lying on your stomach, place a small, flat cushion under your abdomen to support your back. As your abdominals become stronger you should be able to do this exercise without the cushion.

If you have a history of sciatica leave the legs parallel.

There are two stages to this exercise.

## Stage One (beginners)

**Starting Position**

Lie on your front. Have your feet hip-width apart and turned out from the hips (see note above). Rest your forehead on your folded arms. Relax and open the upper body.

**Action**

1 Breathe in to prepare and lengthen through the spine.
2 Breathe out, zip up and hollow, and stay zipped throughout. First lengthen, then raise one leg lifting it no more than five centimetres off the ground.
3 Lengthen away from a strong centre. Do not twist in the pelvis; both hip joints stay on the floor. Try to keep your shoulders relaxed and a sense of width in your upper body.
4 Breathe in, lengthen and lower the leg.
5 Repeat eight times with each leg.

**Watchpoints**

* Keep the lower abdominals supporting your lower back.
* Think of creating space round the hip joint as you lengthen the leg away.
* Be careful to keep both hip joints on the floor – you are only lifting the leg.
* Don't let the pelvis roll or twist, keep it square.
* Keep your neck long and relaxed, the head stays down on the floor throughout the exercise.
* Everyone lifts the legs too high, only lift it just a few centimetres.

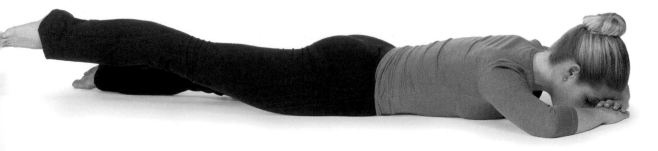

# Stage Two (intermediate)

## Equipment
A folded towel or flat cushion (optional).

## Starting Position
Lie on your front with your feet hip-width apart. Take your arms out just wider than shoulder-width, so that you look like a star. Remember good upper-body use: your shoulder blades do not rise up round your ears, there is distance between the ears and the shoulders. Keep a sense of openness in the upper body. You may like to place a small very flat cushion or folded towel under your forehead. You want the neck to be in a neutral position with a natural curve to the neck, not squashed backwards or forwards.

## Action
1 Breathe in to prepare and lengthen through the spine.
2 Breathe out, zip up and hollow, and stay zipped throughout. Lengthen first, then simultaneously raise the opposite arm and leg no more than five centimetres off the ground. Allow your head to lift with the arm movement, but remember to keep the back of the neck long, stay looking down. Lengthen away from a strong centre.
3 Do not twist in the pelvis; both hip joints stay on the floor. Try to keep a sense of width in your upper body.
4 Breathe in and relax.
5 Repeat with the opposite side.
6 Repeat five times on each side.

## Watchpoints
• As for Stage One.
• Do not overreach or over-lift the arms. Keep the elbows slightly bent and keep them wide.
• Keep your neck long and relaxed, the head stays down on the floor throughout the exercise.

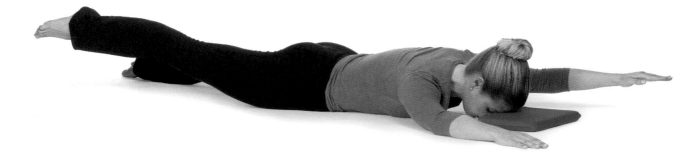

# Star Circles

You will feel this deep in the buttock.

**Starting Position**

As for the Star Stage One (page 75).

**Action**

1  Follow Action Points 1–3 from the Star Stage One, (page 75) turning the leg out from the hip joint, then slowly draw five small circles with the whole leg. The circles should be no bigger than a grapefruit.

2  Breathe in as you circle five times one way and breathe out as your circle five times the opposite way.

**Watchpoints**

•  Keep the hips on the floor and the pelvis still.

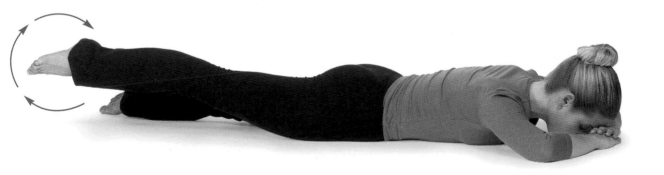

# Front Leg Pull  (*advanced*)

A challenging exercise that requires good upper-body strength as well as good core strength.

## Aim

This exercise really challenges the powerhouse, and conditions the whole body.

## Starting Position

Adopt a traditional push-up position, making sure that your body is long and the shoulders are drawn down into your back. The fingers point forward, the elbows stay straight but not locked, head in line with the body, legs hip-width apart. You should feel as if your body is being pulled in two directions.

**Warning:** avoid this exercise if you have shoulder problems.

## Action

1  Breathe in to prepare.
2  Breathe out and zip up and hollow. Stay zipped throughout, and press the heels away from you. Think of a plank of wood or an ironing board.
3  Breathe in as you lift one leg (keeping the foot flexed) towards the ceiling without moving the hips or allowing the back to arch. Keep lengthening the head away and keep the ribcage flat.
4  Breathe out as you lower the leg back to the floor still lengthening through the heel.
5  Repeat five times with each leg.

## Watchpoints

• Keep your shoulder blades connected down into your back.
• Keep the back of the neck long and released.
• Don't dip in the middle.

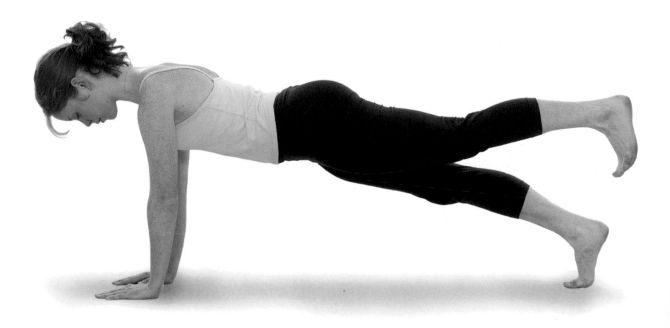

# Rest Position

This is a lovely way to stretch out the back, especially after doing back extensions or four-point kneeling exercises.

Avoid the Rest Position if you have knee problems as you may compress the joint. You may like to have a cushion under the knees.

**Equipment**
A cushion (optional).

**Action**
1 Usually this exercise follows one in which you have been lying prone (on your front). So come up on to all fours, bringing your feet together but keeping your knees apart.
2 Slowly move back towards your buttocks. Do not raise your head or hands and come back to sit on your feet – not between them – the back is rounded.

3 Rest and relax into this position, leave the arms extended to give you a maximum stretch. Feel the expansion of the back of your ribcage as you breathe deeply into it.
4 The further apart the knees are the more of a stretch you will feel in your inner thighs. With the knees in this position, you can really think of your chest sinking down into the floor.
5 You can also have the knees together which stretches out the lumbar spine. We do not recommend this version for anyone with back injuries because it takes the lumbar spine into a very flexed position.
6 Take ten breaths in this position.

**To Come Out of the Rest Position**
1 As you breathe out, zip up and hollow, and slowly unfurl.
2 Think of dropping your tailbone down and bringing your pubic bone forward.
3 Rebuild your spine vertebra by vertebra until you are upright.

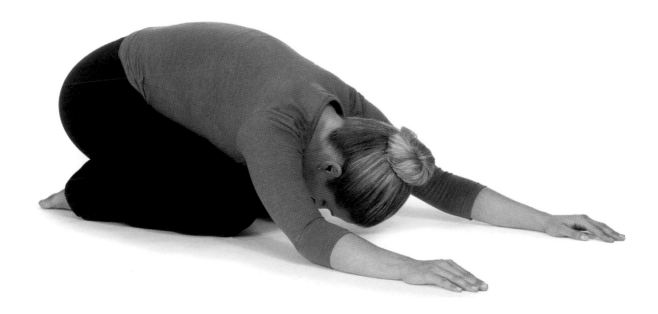

# Sitting Side Reach

A gentle side stretch which feels really good.

We all have a preferred way of sitting cross-legged. It helps to balance the body if you sometimes cross your legs the other way.

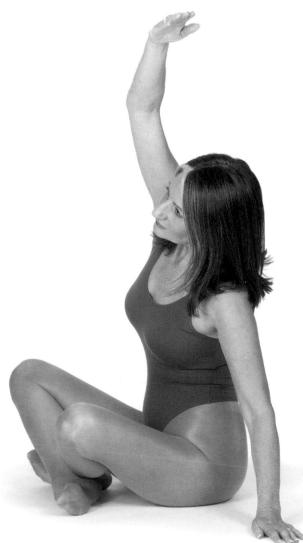

**Equipment**

A rolled-up towel (optional).

**Starting Position**

Sit with a rolled-up towel under your bottom if this is more comfortable. Sit tall with your legs crossed. Make sure you are sitting on your sitting bones and that the natural curves of the spine are maintained. Rest your arms on the floor beside you.

**Action**

1  Breathe in wide to prepare and lengthen up through the spine.
2  Breathe out, zip up and hollow, and stay zipped throughout. Float one arm up, remembering what you learnt in Floating Arms (page 49).
3  Breathe in, then out, and reach up and across, lifting up out of the waist rather than simply reaching through the shoulders. Keep both buttocks firmly on the mat.
4  Breathe in and return to centre.
5  Breathe out and float the arm back down.
6  Repeat twice to each side, then change the way you are sitting cross-legged and repeat twice more to each side.

**Watchpoints**

• Try not to lean forward or back, but go directly to the side.
• Keep your head in a line with your spine.

# Sitting Twist

Another simple cross-legged exercise. Sit on a rolled up towel if you prefer. This time we want to achieve a gentle rotation in the spine. Although this is a very simple exercise it feels really good, especially between the shoulder blades. Experiment with the breathing to see if you prefer to twist on an in or an out breath.

**Equipment**

A rolled-up towel (optional).

**Starting Position**

Sit tall, crossed-legged, with your weight evenly balanced on both sitting bones.

**Action**

1 Breathe in and lengthen up through the spine. Place your right hand on your left knee and your left hand behind you.
2 Breathe out, zip up and hollow, and stay zipped throughout. Slowly turn your torso and head so you are looking over your shoulder. Try to feel each vertebra rotating on its neighbour, so that you feel the twist deep in the spine. Don't turn the head too far; it stays in a line with the spine.
3 Breathe normally. Try to soften between the shoulder blades – this is where we hold tension. Keep the shoulders down and the neck released. Keep lengthening up.
4 After four breaths, slowly return to the centre.
5 Repeat three times to each side. Experiment with twisting on the in breath to see which suits you better.

**Watchpoints**

• Keep your weight evenly balanced on both sitting bones.
• Don't sink down, but keep lengthening up.
• Do not push on the hand resting on the knee – it is just there to guide you, not turn you further around.

# Arm Openings

This has to be the most relaxing, feel-good exercise in the Pilates programme. If you stay completely aware of your arm and hand as they displace the air moving through space, you will achieve a sense of openness while stabilizing and centring. This exercise will also open the upper body and stretch the pectoral muscles, while gently and safely rotating the spine.

**Equipment**

A plump cushion.
A tennis ball (optional).

**Starting Position**

Lie on your side with your head on a cushion and your knees curled up at a right angle to your body. Your back should be in a 'straight' line, but with its natural curve. You may place a tennis ball between the knees (the idea is for the tennis ball to keep your knees and pelvis is good alignment). Align all your bones: feet, ankles, knees, hips and shoulders, and extend your arms in front of you, palms together, at shoulder height.

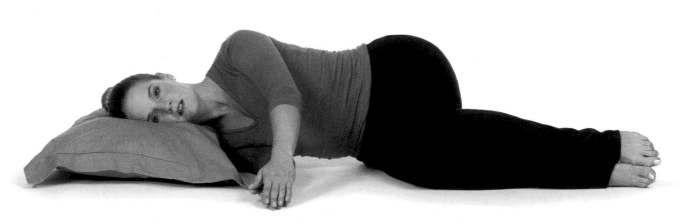

## Action

1 Breathe in to prepare, and lengthen through the spine.
2 Breathe out, zip up and hollow, and stay zipped throughout.
3 Breathe in as you slowly extend and lift the upper arm, keeping the elbow soft and the shoulder blade down into the back. Keep your eyes on your hand so that the head follows the arm movement. You are aiming to touch the floor behind you, but do not force it.
4 Try to keep your knees together and your pelvis still.
5 Breathe out as you bring the arm back in an arc to rest on the other hand again.
6 Repeat five times, then curl up on the other side and start again.

## Watchpoints

• Keep hollowing throughout.
• Keep your waist long and lifted – don't allow it to sink into the floor.
• Allow your head to roll naturally with the movement, make sure that the cushion supports it.
• Keep the gap between your ears and your shoulders by engaging the muscles below the shoulder blades.

**Warning:** as this exercise involves rotation of the spine, take advice if you have a disc-related injury.

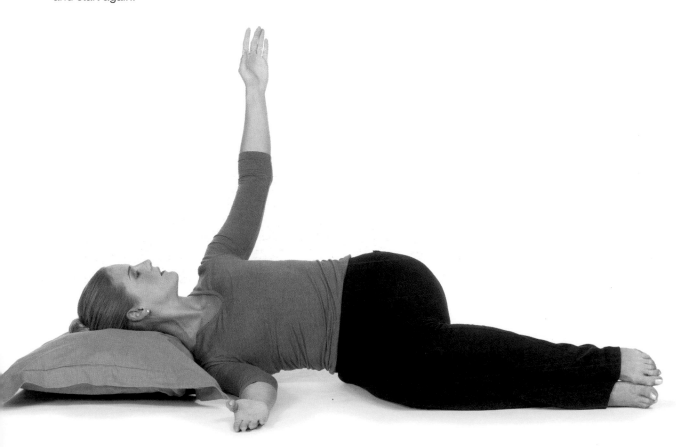

# Hip Rolls  (*beginners*)

This exercise works the waist muscles, but also teaches you how to rotate the spine safely with stability and length. The tennis ball ensures that you keep good alignment of the knees and hips.

Please take advice if you have a disc-related injury.

## Equipment
A tennis ball.

## Starting Position
Lie in the Relaxation Position (page 31), and bring your feet together, lining up the bones. Put the tennis ball between your knees. Place your arms out to the sides just below shoulder height, palms down.

## Action
1  Breathe in wide and full to prepare.
2  Breathe out, zip up and hollow, and stay zipped throughout. Roll your head in one direction, your knees in the other. Only roll a little way to start with – you can go further each time if it is comfortable. Keep your opposite shoulder down on the floor. Your feet stay glued together moving with the legs (see Watchpoints).

3  Breathe in.
4  Breathe out, and use your strong centre to bring the knees back to the Starting Position; the head comes back as well.
5  Repeat eight times in each direction. Think of rolling each part of your back off the floor in sequence and then returning the back of the ribcage, the waist, the small of your back, the buttock in that order to the floor.

## Watchpoints
• Your feet will make an action a bit like an aeroplane banking. They do not stay flat on the floor, but the side of one foot always stays in contact with it.
• Keep working those abdominals. Do not simply allow the weight of the legs to pull you over.

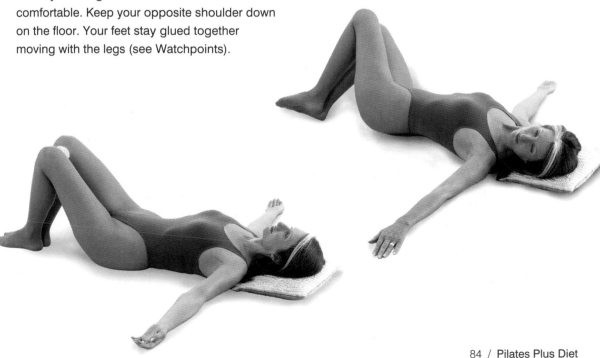

# Kneeling Hip Flexor Stretch

If you needed proof that your alignment is key when trying to isolate certain muscles, this is the exercise to provide it. To feel the stretch at the front of the hip, you need to position your body correctly and then make only the slightest movement – no need to make giant lunges forward, the movement is very subtle.

**Aim**
To stretch the hip flexors.

**Starting Position**
Kneel on your mat. Take your right leg out in front of you in a line with your hip joint. Place the foot flat on the mat and have the leg bent so that the knee forms a 90° angle and is directly over the ankle. Your left leg and foot should also be in a line with your left hip. Check that your pelvis is square and facing forward. Both sides of the waist should be equally long.

**Action**
1  Breathe in wide and lengthen up through the spine.
2  Breathe out and zip up and hollow. Very gently drop your tailbone down, tucking under (that is tilt the pelvis to north, see the Compass on page 39). Breathe normally and see if you can feel a stretch at the front of the left hip (the stretch may go down into the front of the thigh). If you cannot feel the stretch, tuck under a little more or try moving the pelvis forward a fraction (as if you are thrusting through!). This is a very individual thing, everyone feels the stretch slightly differently.
3  Hold this position for a few breaths. Keep lengthening upwards.
4  Repeat three times on each side.

**Watchpoints**
• Make sure that your front knee doesn't move over the foot, keep it directly above the ankle.
• Think about your upper body; shoulder blades rest down into the back.

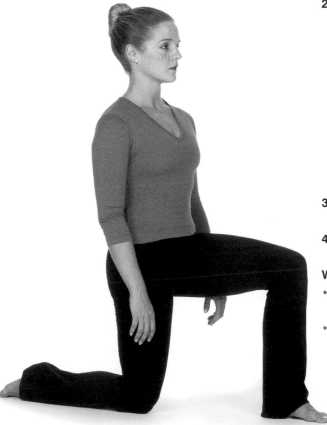

# Monkey Bends

A subtle exercise that works on lengthening your spine and strengthening your postural muscles and legs.

### Starting Position
Stand tall, feet hip-width apart and in parallel. Place your hands on the front of your thighs.

### Action
1 Breathe in wide, and lengthen through the top of your head.
2 Breathe out, zip up and hollow, and stay zipped throughout. Bend your knees directly over the centre of each foot, simultaneously hingeing forward and pivoting from the hip joint.
3 Slide your hands down your thighs. Keep your back long and in one piece with the head and neck. Think of the top of your head lengthening away from your tailbone.
4 Breathe in and lengthen back up to standing tall.
5 Repeat six times.

### Watchpoints
* Keep your weight evenly distributed between both feet.
* Keep the back of the neck long, your neck released.

**Variation:** Monkey Bends with Shoulder Reach (all levels).

### Starting Position
As for Monkey Bends.

### Action
1 Follow Action points 1 and 2 above, but this time raise both arms to shoulder height as if doing Shoulder Reaches (page 47)
2 Breathe in and lower the arms, lengthening back up to standing tall.

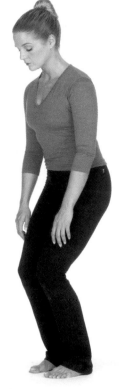
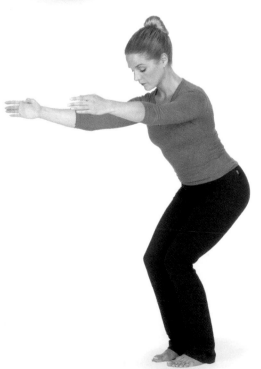

# Demi-Pliés in Turn Out

A lot of Pilates exercises have a ballet influence –
they are great for building muscle in the body
especially on the inner thighs and buttocks.

## Starting Position

Stand tall, side-on to the wall or a chair. Put your
hand on the wall to help your balance. Turn your
legs out from the hip joints. It's very important that
you do not just turn out from the knees or ankles –
the action comes from the hips.

## Action

1  Breathe in wide and lengthen through the spine.
2  Breathe out, zip up and hollow, and stay zipped
   throughout. Bend the knees over the centre of
   the toes. Keep the heels down and try not to
   tip forward.
3  Breathe in and slowly straighten your legs,
   pulling up through the inner thighs and
   squeezing the buttocks. Feel that you are
   turning out from deep in the hips.
4  Repeat eight times.

## Watchpoints

* Keep good alignment through the body.
* Use your core muscles to keep
  you centred.
* Feel as though you are being pulled
  up right through your body from
  your heels, up the inner thighs,
  through the spine and through
  the top of the head.

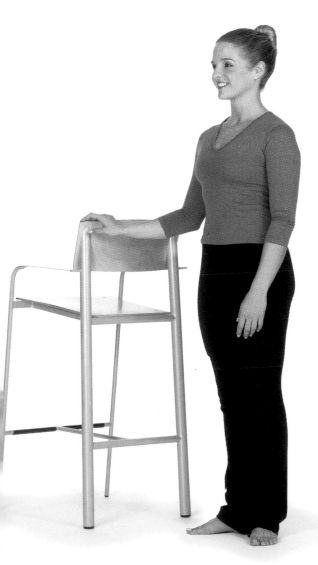
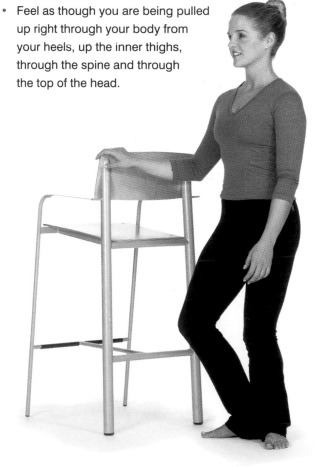

# Up and Down Barre Exercise

This wonderful exercise can be done anywhere. It strengthens the legs and buttocks, teaches good postural alignment, strengthens and stretches the calf muscles and works the deep calf pump thus improving the circulation in the legs.

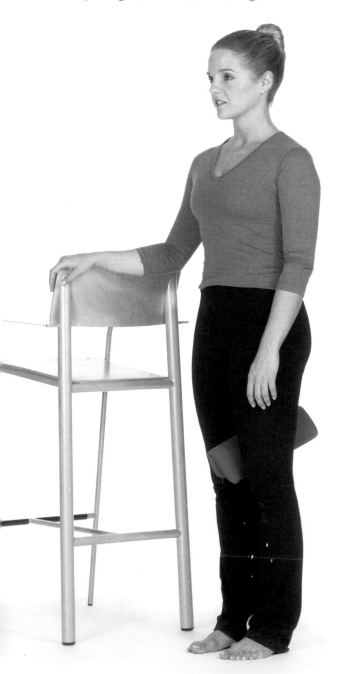

## Equipment
A tennis ball.
Another tennis ball or a small cushion.

## Starting Position
Stand side-on to a wall or next to the back of a chair, and place the tennis ball between your ankles, just below your ankle bone. Place another tennis ball or a small cushion between the thighs, just above the knees. Stand well (see Standing Correctly on page 32) and put your hand on the wall or the chair to help you balance.

## Action
1  Breathe in and lengthen up through the spine – imagine someone is pulling you up from the top of your head, but that there is also a weight on your tailbone, anchoring your spine.
2  Breathe out and zip up and hollow. Rise up on to your toes.
3  Breathe in.
4  Breathe out, and slowly lengthen your heels back down on the floor away from the top of your head. Imagine that your head stays up there.
5  When your heels are on the floor, bend your knees slightly directly over your feet, keeping the heels down. Do not allow your bottom to stick out.
6  Repeat ten times.

## Watchpoints
• Do not allow your bottom to stick out as you bend the knees.
• Keep the heels on the ground as you bend the knees.
• Keep the weight evenly balanced on the feet.
• Keep lengthening upwards throughout.

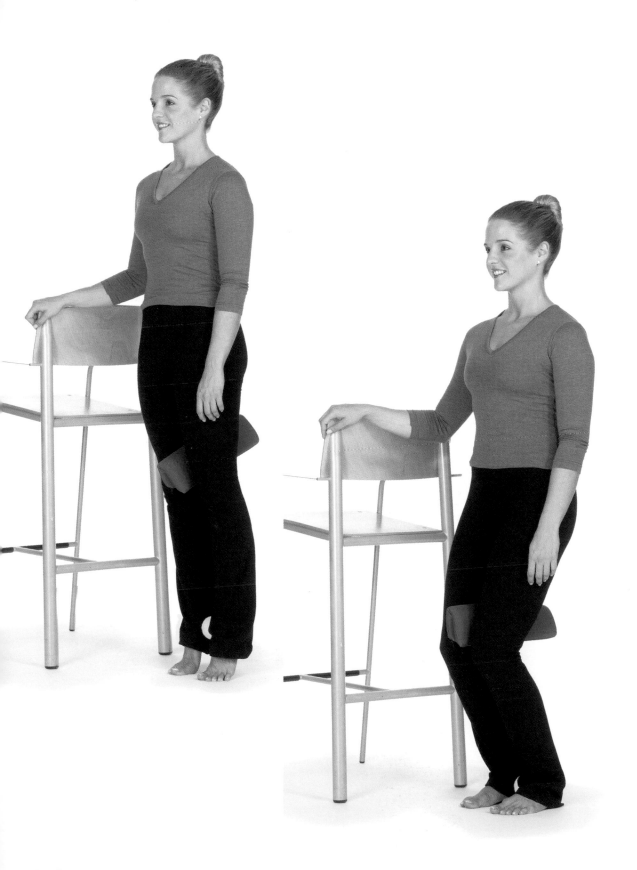

# Up and Down on One Leg

This has all the benefits of the previous exercise, but because your weight is now on one leg, it is weight bearing and thus more strengthening. You will not really feel this exercise working until you have done about four repetitions, and then you will feel which muscles you are working – honestly!

**Starting Position**

Stand side-on to a wall or the back of a chair. Put a hand on the wall or chair to help you balance. Take one foot off the floor.

**Action**

1 Breathe in and lengthen up through the spine – imagine someone is pulling you up from the top of your head, but that there is also a weight on your tailbone, anchoring your spine.
2 Breathe out, zip up and hollow, and rise up on your toes.
3 Breathe in.
4 Breathe out, and slowly lengthen your heels back down on the floor away from the top of your head. Imagine that your head stays up there.
5 When your heel is on the floor, slightly bend your knee directly over your foot, keeping the heel down. Do not allow your bottom to stick out.
6 Repeat ten times with each leg.

**Watchpoints**

* Keep both sides of your waist long and your pelvis level. Do not sink into one hip.
* Keep thinking up, up, up.
* Keep the heel on the ground as you bend the knee.
* Keep lengthening upwards throughout.

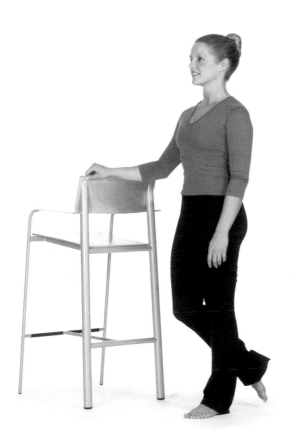

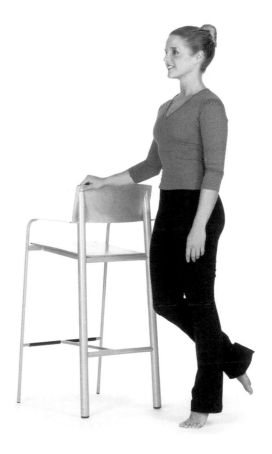

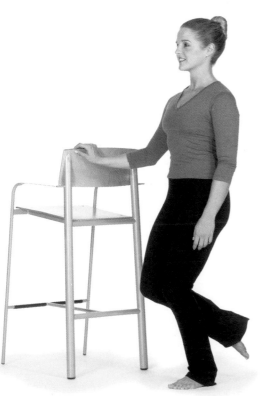

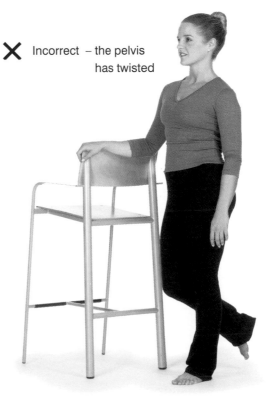

✗ Incorrect – the pelvis
has twisted

The Exercises

# Side-lying Front and Back (*intermediate*)

**Equipment**

A flat cushion (optional).

**Starting Position**

Lie on your side in a straight line. Using the edge of your mat as a guide, stack all the joints on top of each other: shoulder over shoulder, hip over hip, knee over knee. Your natural spine curves are maintained. Bring both legs in front of you to an angle of about 45° (you may need to vary this – you should feel stable). The upper arm is on the floor in line with your body and the elbow is bent. You can either stretch the lower arm out in a line with the body, and rest your head on a flat cushion positioned between the ear and the outstretched arm, or, rest your head in your hand with the elbow bent in a line with your shoulder. Do not roll the body forward. Imagine a wall behind your body; keep in contact with that wall with both shoulders.

**Action**

1  Breathe in and lengthen through the whole body.
2  Breathe out, zip up and hollow, and stay zipped throughout. Bring the top leg up to hip height and point the toe.
3  Breathe in and swing the leg forward. Do not allow the back to round or arch. The torso stays still.
4  Breathe out and swing the leg back. Take it behind you, but do not allow the back to arch or the hips to push forward.
5  Breathe in and swing the leg forward.
6  Repeat six times on each side.

**Watchpoints**

* Keep your torso still – use the powerhouse muscles.
* Keep lengthening through the spine, don't collapse in the middle.
* Keep the leg hip height off the floor and the leg in parallel, not turned in or out.
* Do not allow the back to arch as the leg comes back.

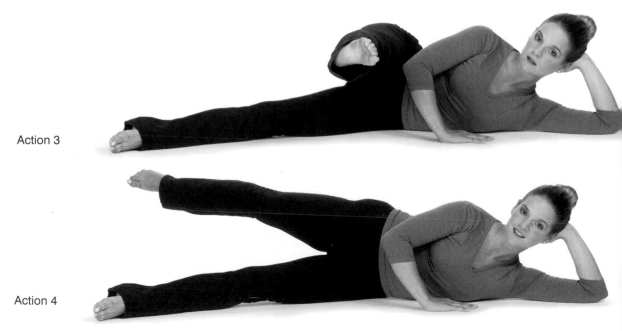

Action 3

Action 4

# Side-lying Bicycles (*advanced*)

This exercise works the leg and buttock muscles, as well as strengthening your core powerhouse muscles.

Keep the upper body still throughout the exercise. Do not allow the waist to sink into the floor. Notice a change in breathing pattern once the exercise gets going!

**Starting Position**
As for Side-lying Front and Back on page 92.

**Action**

1  Breathe in wide and lengthen through the whole body. Keep the waist long.
2  Breathe out, zip up and hollow, and stay zipped throughout. Raise and bend the top knee in towards your chest keeping it at hip height.
3  Breathe in and slowly straighten the leg in front of you. Flex the foot.

4  Breathe out and bring the leg back until it is in a line with your body. Then, if you can, point the foot and take the leg behind you, without arching the back or pushing the hips forward.
5  Breathe in and slowly bend the knee in, then straighten it in front of you. Flex the foot.
6  Breathe out and sweep the leg back (see Action 4, opposite). Point the foot.
7  Repeat five times on each side.

**Watchpoints**

*  Keep your torso still – use the powerhouse muscles.
*  Don't collapse in the middle.
*  Keep the leg hip height off the floor and parallel, not turned in or out.
*  Do not allow the back to arch as the leg comes back.
*  Keep the actions smooth, continuous and flowing – like riding a bike!

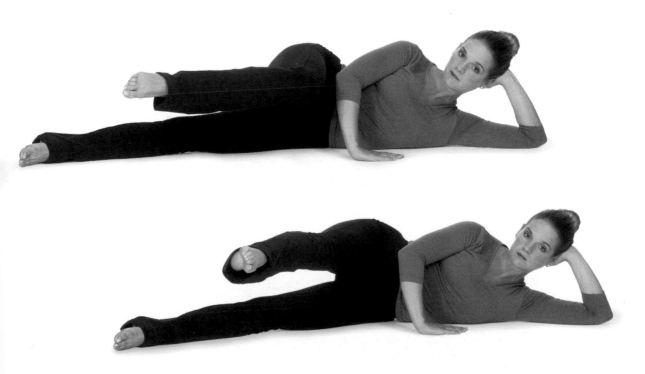

# The Torpedo  (*intermediate*)

This side-lying exercise really works the waist.

**Equipment**
A flat cushion (optional).

**Starting Position**
Lie on your side in a straight line, stacking your
joints on top of each other. Have your lower arm
stretched out in a line with your body. Rest your
head on your outstretched arm (you may use a flat
cushion if you wish). Place your uppermost arm in
front of you in a line with your chest, palm flat,
fingertips pointing away from your feet.

**Action**
1   Breathe out, zip up and hollow, and stay
    zipped throughout.
2   Breathe in and lift both legs up together in
    a straight line with your body.
3   Breathe out and raise the upper leg slightly
    higher, keeping it parallel to the lower leg.
    The lower leg stays up. Feel the length of the
    body from fingertip to toes, long and strong.
4   Breathe in and lower the top leg to the
    bottom leg.
5   Breathe out and gently lower both legs back
    to the floor.
6   Repeat five times to each side.

**Watchpoints**
•   Try not to use your supporting arm to push
    yourself up.
•   Make sure you maintain neutral pelvis and spine.
    Do not arch the back.
•   The elbow of the supporting arm stays open.
    The shoulder stays down.
•   Really enjoy lengthening through the whole body.

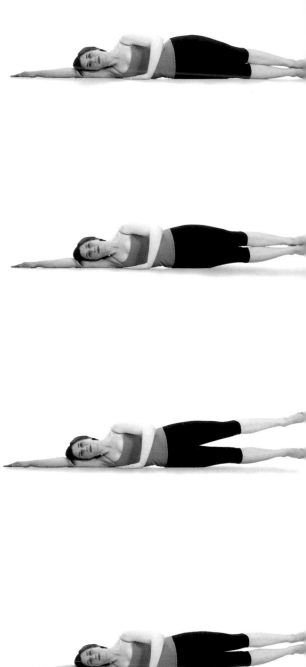

# Arm Circles with Weights  (*intermediate*)

A great exercise for strengthening the arms and shoulders. Try it first without the weights to perfect your technique.

**Equipment**
Hand-held weights of 0.5kg each weight.

**Starting Position**
Lie in the Relaxation Position (page 31). Have your arms down by your side, palms facing down.

**Action**

1 Breathe in wide and full. Lengthen through the body.
2 Breathe out, zip up and hollow, and stay zipped throughout. Raise your arms up. Take them behind you a few centimetres off the floor.
3 Breathe in as you circle them out to the sides and back down, bending your elbows slightly. Turn the palms down as you reach your sides. Keep your arms off the floor.
4 Repeat five times, then reverse the direction of the circle and repeat another five times.

**Watchpoints**

• Maintain neutral pelvis and spine throughout and do not allow the upper back to arch.
• Do not allow the ribs to flare. Move with the breath.
• Keep the shoulder blades wide and down the back, but do allow for mobility; no gripping!
• Keep the neck long and released.
• Watch the alignment of the hands and wrists!
• Keep the elbows soft.

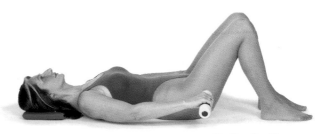

Starting Position.

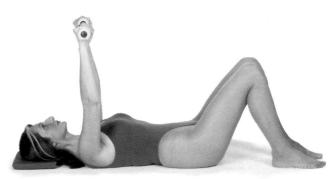

Action 2

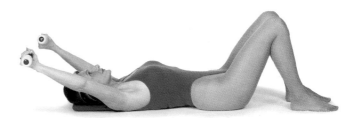

Action 3

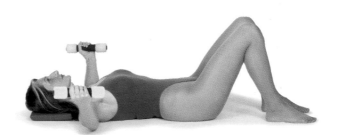

Action 4

# Arm Weights: Triceps

There are many ways to work the triceps. This one is great because there is no risk of over-using your neck muscles. You will need to take a firm grip on the weight. We have added a cushion squeeze here as well, so that you work your inner thighs at the same time.

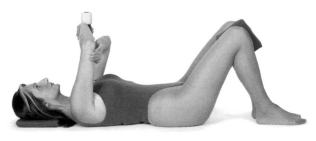

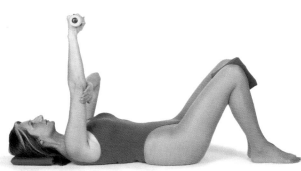

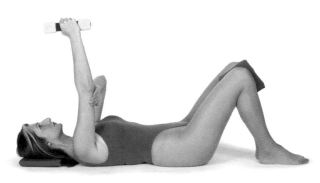

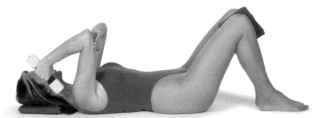

## Equipment

A hand-held weight up to 2.5kg. You can either buy a long hand-held weight or use a tall can or a heavy rolling pin. (You may use heavier weights if you wish to sculpt the arms.)

A cushion.

## Starting Position

Lie with your knees bent and your pelvis in neutral. Place a small cushion between your knees and throughout the exercise you squeeze the cushion to work the inner thighs. Hold the weight in one hand so that your palm faces away from you, your knuckles towards you. The wrist is in a line with the forearm. Your elbow is bent directly over your shoulder. Your upper arm is vertical to you. Angle the lower part of the arm so that your hand could touch your opposite shoulder.

## Action

1 Breathing normally throughout, slowly straighten your arm, keeping the elbow quite still. Do not fully straighten the arm, stop just short.
2 Then turn your arm so that the palm faces inwards.
3 Bring the hand down so it almost touches the same shoulder.
4 Straighten the arm, turn and bend it again, so you almost touch the opposite shoulder. This way you work both the triceps and the biceps. Keep your upper arm still.
5 Repeat up to twenty times with each arm.

## Watchpoints

* Keep your neck released and your shoulder blades down into your back
* If you are squeezing the cushion between your knees, be sure that you do not tilt the pelvis or grip around the hips.

# Standing Tarzan

A fun exercise in the standing weights series.
It targets the biceps.

## Equipment
Light hand-held weights up to 1kg each weight.

## Starting Position
Stand correctly (page 32). Hold your arms out to the sides, palms facing upwards holding the weights, shoulder blades down into your back, neck released. Have the arms straight but not locked.

## Action
1 Breathe in wide and full, and lengthen up through the spine.
2 Breathe out, zip up and hollow, and stay gently zipped throughout. Slowly curl your arms in, hingeing from the elbows.
3 Breathe in and slowly straighten the arm again.
4 Repeat eight times.

## Watchpoints
• Keep the upper arm quite still.
• As you straighten the arms think of lengthening away.

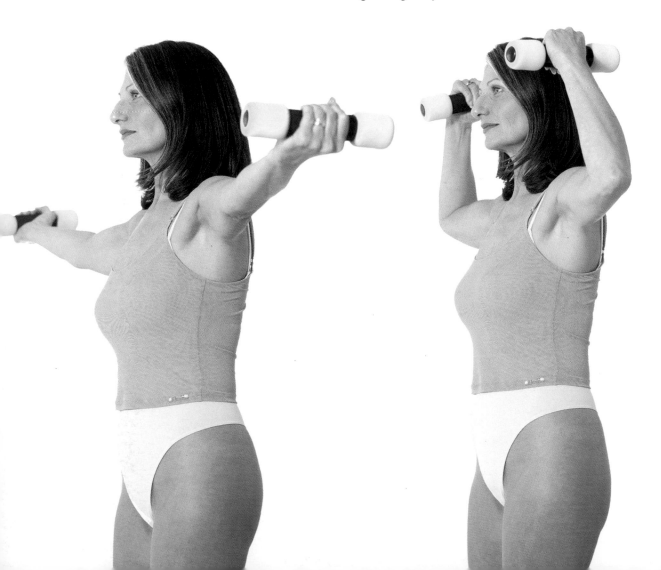

# Arm Pulls

You feel this one deep in the upper arm and armpit area. Focus on both lifting and lowering the weights very slowly and with control.

## Equipment
Hand-held weights up to 1kg each weight.

## Starting Position
Stand correctly (page 32). Hold the weights down in front of you, the weights just touching, palms facing the body.

## Action
1 Breathe in wide and lengthen through the spine.
2 Breathe out, zip up and hollow, and stay zipped throughout. Lift the weights along an imaginary line up the centre of your body to about nipple height. Make sure you use your arms to do the work; the shoulders stay down into your back.
3 Breathe in and slowly lower.
4 Repeat ten times.

## Watchpoints
• Keep the wrists strong.
• Maintain the distance between your ears and your shoulders.
• Keep the upper body wide and open.
• Keep your neck released.

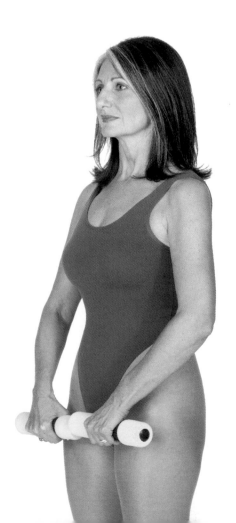
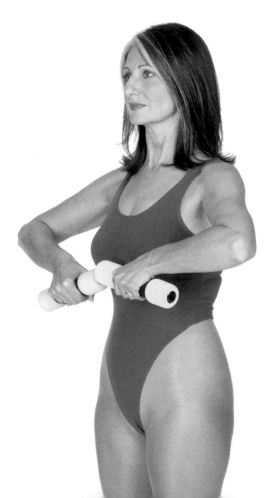

# Back Press with Weights

Opens the chest and strengthens the mid-back muscles and the core muscles, which have to keep good alignment. Keeping good alignment through the body is essential in this exercise. It is very easy to tip the upper body forward. Use your core muscles to keep you upright, head balanced over ribcage, over pelvis, over released knees. Weight even on the centre of the feet – don't rock forward or back.

**Equipment**
Hand-held weights of 0.5kg each weight.

**Starting Position**
Stand correctly (page 32) with your arms relaxed down by your sides, palms facing backwards. Hold a weight in each hand.

**Action**
1 Breathe in wide and lengthen through the spine
2 Breathe out and zip up and hollow.
3 Breathe in and press your arms back, opening the chest but not allowing the upper back to arch or the ribcage to flare.
4 Breathe out and bring the arms back.
5 Repeat six times.

**Watchpoints**
• Keep your neck released.
• Try not to squeeze between the shoulder blades
• Keep the distance between your ears and your shoulders.

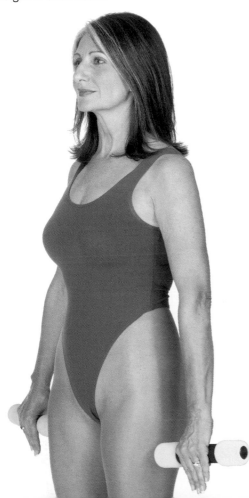
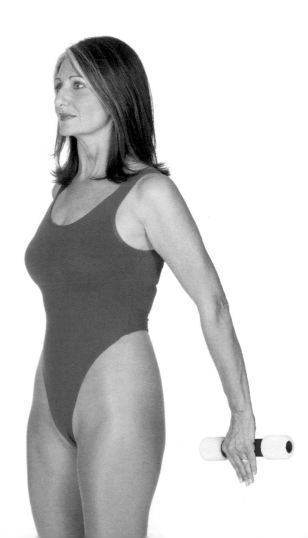

# Roll Downs with Weights  (*beginners/intermediate*)

This is a real feel-good exercise which works the postural muscles. It combines stabilizing work with the wonderful wheeling motion of the spine.

As you roll back up, think of rebuilding the spinal column, stacking each vertebra on top of the other to lengthen out the spine.

We have added an extra element with the optional use of hand weights – they increase the sense of release in the upper body and help build muscles.

**Equipment**
Hand-held weights 0.5kg each weight.

**Starting Position**
Stand with your feet hip-width apart and in parallel, your weight evenly balanced on both feet. Check that you are not rolling your feet in or out. Soften your knees. Find your neutral pelvis position but keep the tailbone lengthening down. Hold the weights in each hand if you are using them.

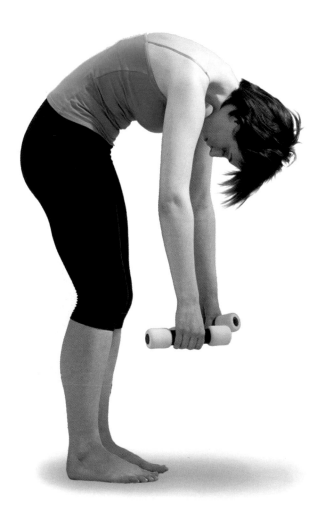

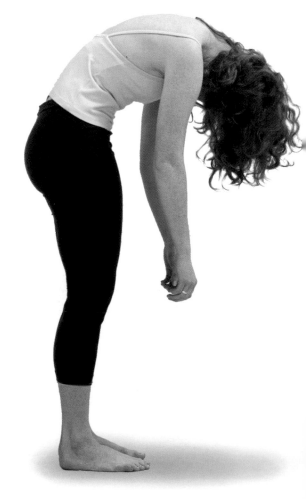

## Action

1 Breathe in to prepare and lengthen through the spine. Release the head and neck.
2 Breathe out, zip up and hollow, and stay zipped throughout. Drop your chin down to your chest and allow the weight of your head to make you roll slowly forward, head released, arms hanging, centre strong, knees soft.
3 Breathe in as you hang, really letting your head and arms hang.
4 Breathe out, firmly zipped, as you drop your tailbone down. Directing your pubic bone forward, rotate your pelvis backwards as you slowly come up to standing tall, rolling through the spine bone by bone.
5 Repeat six times.

## Watchpoints

• You may like to take an extra breath during the exercise. This is fine, but please try to breathe out as you move the spine.
• Make sure that you go down centrally and you do not sway over to one side. When you are down, check where your hands are in relation to your feet.
• Do not roll the feet in or out. Keep the weight evenly balanced and try not to lean forward on to the front of your feet or back on to the heels.
• As you come up to standing tall, think of your shoulder blade connection.

Warning: please take advice if you have a back problem, especially if disc-related.

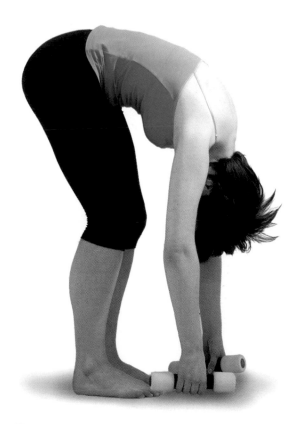
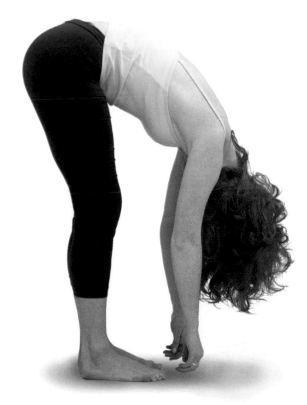

# Abductor Lifts/Outer Thigh Toner  (*intermediate*)

These two exercises really target the thigh muscles and work the waist.

Practise them firstly without weights, until you are totally familiar with them and they cause you no discomfort.

### Equipment
Leg weights (opitional) of up to 1.5 kg. strapped on to your ankles. Start with the lightest weight.

A cushion (optional).

### Starting Position
Lie on your left side in a straight line – this is crucial, so, if you like, you can lie up against a wall to check your alignment. Don't lean on the wall! Your left arm is stretched out; your head rests on the arm. You may place a cushion between your ear and your arm so that the head is at the correct angle to the spine. Bend both legs in front of you at an angle of just under 90°. Put your right hand in front of your body to help support you. Throughout the exercise, keep lifting the waist off the floor and maintaining the length in the trunk.

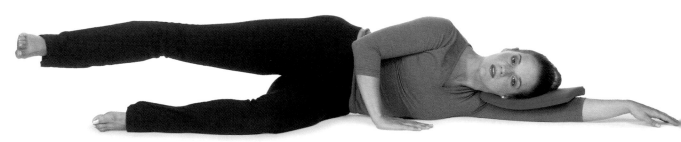

**Action**

1   Zip up and hollow, and stay zipped throughout. Straighten your top leg so it is in a line with your hip and about twelve centimetres off the floor. Be careful not to take it behind you! Softly flex the foot towards your face.
2   Breathe out as you slowly lift the leg about fifteen centimetres, then breathe in and lower.
3   Raise and lower the leg ten times, without returning it to the floor. You are breathing out as you raise, and in as you lower.
4   Bend the leg to rest on the bent one underneath.
5   Repeat ten times, then rest a few seconds and do ten more repetitions. Do the Inner Thigh Toner on page 104 before you do the other side.

**Watchpoints**

•   Keep zipping and hollowing so that you protect the low back and prevent it from arching, or the waist from dropping down to the floor.
•   Lengthen the heel as far away as possible from the hip – long, long leg.
•   Keep lifting the waist off the floor and lengthening in the body – long, long waist.
•   Your pelvis should remain absolutely still; do not allow it to roll forward or rock around.
•   Don't forget to keep the upper body open and your shoulder blades down into your back. Do not allow yourself to roll forward.

If you are lucky enough to lack any natural padding round your hip, you may find it uncomfortable to lie like this. If so, just put a small piece of foam underneath your hip.

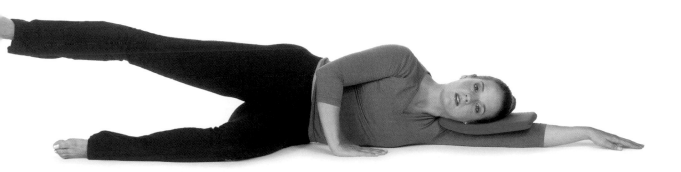

# Inner Thigh Toner  (*intermediate*)

It does what it says – tones the adductors!

## Equipment
As for Abductor Lifts (page 102).
    A plump cushion.

## Starting Position
Lie on your left side as for Abductor Lifts (page 102) but bend your top knee and rest it on top of a large cushion. The idea is for your pelvis to stay square and not drop forward. Stretch the bottom leg away a little in front of you, turning it out from the hip joint. Point or flex the foot, either is fine.

## Action
1 Breathe in wide and full to prepare.
2 Keeping the leg turned out from the hip, long and straight, breathe out, zip up and hollow, and stay zipped throughout. Slowly raise the underneath leg. Keep lengthening it away. Do not allow your waist to sink into the floor, keep working it.
3 Breathe in as you lower the leg.
4 Repeat ten times, rest a few moments and then do ten more repetitions before turning over and doing the Leg Abductor Lifts and Inner Thigh Toner on the other side.

## Watchpoints
* Keep zipping and hollowing throughout.
* Don't let the waist sag, keep lengthening it.
* Check that you are moving the whole leg together and not just twisting from the knee.

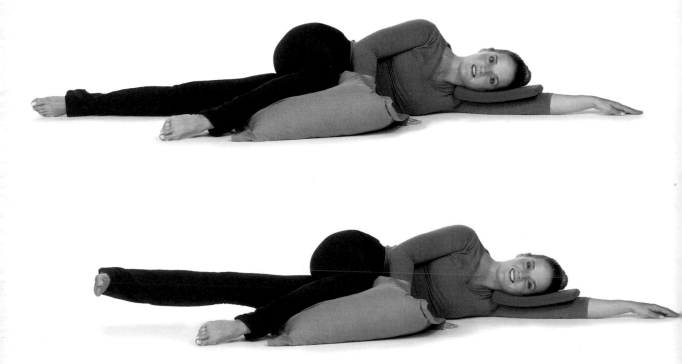

# 4

## The Philosophy Behind
## our Nutritional Approach

# Choosing the Right Diet

**Losing weight is easy** – it's keeping it off that's the real challenge. The sad fact is that most people who lose weight end up regaining it. Why? Because most diets provide a short-term fix to what is a long-term problem.

Don't think about dieting as a short-term solution. The only way to lose weight safely and permanently is to make long-term changes in your food choices, eating habits and lifestyle. So forget about dieting and start thinking about a whole new way of eating. This doesn't mean you have to miss out on your favourite foods – in fact it's important to include the foods you enjoy eating. A diet that leaves you feeling deprived, unhappy and dissatisfied, is a diet that's going to be abandoned.

# The Diet Myth

How often have you been tempted by the promise of losing 7 kilos in 7 days, only to find that the very next week you've regained all the weight you lost, plus a little more? Yo-yo dieting – repeatedly losing and regaining weight – is not healthy. The best and safest way to lose weight is slowly and steadily – between 0.5–1kg a week is the ideal rate. If you lose too much weight too quickly, there is a danger you will lose lean muscle tissue as well as fat. Since our metabolic rate is related to the amount of lean muscles tissue we have, it's a good idea to preserve it by avoiding unhealthy ways of eating. The following diets promise instant weight loss but do not provide a permanent solution.

**Crash Diets**

Crash diets are not the answer. For every 5 kilos you lose, you'll end up regaining 10 kilos. These diets don't teach you how to change your everyday eating habits, which is what you need to do if you are going to keep the weight off long term.

**Food Combining Diets**

Any eating plan that restricts the amount and type of food you eat results in weight loss. But, there is nothing special about food combining and no scientific reason why it works better than anything else.

**Fad Diets**

These types of diets, such as the Cabbage Soup Diet or the Beverly Hills Diet, are often popular with celebrities, but provide a short-term fix for a problem that needs a long-term solution. They are often lacking in important nutrients.

**Calorie-controlled Ready Meals**

These can be useful to keep in the freezer for times when you don't feel like cooking, but, on the whole, you'd be nutritionally better off making your own meals from fresh ingredients.

**High-fibre Diets**

High-fibre foods are more filling and help you feel full more quickly and stop you feeling hungry for longer. But, large quantities of fibre can hinder the absorption of certain nutrients and can cause uncomfortable bloating in some people.

**Low-fat Diets**

Because fat contains twice as many calories as either protein or carbohydrate, low-fat diets are a very effective way of reducing calorie intake. As fat adds flavour and texture to foods, very low-fat diets can be rather bland and unexciting increasing the likelihood of breaking the diet through sheer boredom.

**Meal Replacement Drinks or Bars**

Fine occasionally if you don't feel like cooking, but real food tastes much better.

# Understanding your Relationship with Food

Before we can understand the complex relationship we have with food we need to understand that we eat for a variety of reasons. We use food to celebrate, to relieve boredom, to make us feel better when we're unhappy or lonely. Certain people, places, moods and situations can also prompt us to eat. Of course, we do eat to satisfy hunger, but often it's to satisfy a psychological rather than a physiological need.

**How to Keep a Food Diary**
Often we're unaware of the external triggers that cause us to eat even when we're not particularly hungry. Keeping a food diary will help you identify them. Keep a record of everything you eat and drink and how you feel for a month. At the end of the month review your diary and make a list of all the triggers that prompt you to eat when you're not really hungry.

Once you've identified the triggers, you can start to think about the ways to avoid those situations.

Using a technique called behaviour modification, you can work out strategies to help you change the way you respond.

If, for instance, when you get home after work you're so hungry you end up eating a family-sized pack of cheesy snacks while preparing the evening meal, plan ahead and have a healthy snack such as a banana or a yoghurt before you leave the office, so you won't be so hungry when you get home.

If your diary reveals that you use food as a way of making yourself feel better when you're unhappy, make a list of non-food related activities that will help lift your spirits when you're feeling low. Rent a movie, have a manicure or take a long, leisurely bath rather than reaching for a chocolate bar. Old habits are hard to break and changing ingrained behaviour patterns is not something you can achieve overnight but, by using behaviour modification techniques, you can teach your body to respond differently.

| Date and time | Where you are | What you're doing/who you're with | How you feel (e.g. tired, unhappy, bored) | What you ate | How hungry are you? On a scale of 1-5* |
|---|---|---|---|---|---|
| Wednesday 3.30pm | Anna's house | Popped round to visit Anna | Ok | 3 chocolate biscuits | 5 not hungry but Anna got the chocolate biscuits out and I couldn't resist |
| Thursday 10.30am | In the office | Work | Fine | Chocolate bar | 2 skipped breakfast so I feel quite hungry |
| Thursday 10pm | At home | By myself watching TV | Bored/tired – late back from work, no energy to make proper meal | Half a tube of Pringles and bottle of white wine | 1 starving after a long day at work |
| | | | | | 1=hungry / 5=not hungry |

# 5

## The Daily Meal Planner

# How the Diet Plan Works

- Drink a large glass of water, either still or sparkling, before each meal.

- Drink 150ml unsweetened fruit juice for breakfast every day.

- Vegetables and salad are allowed freely so make the most of them – have at least one serving with each meal.

- Include a piece of fresh fruit or a fresh fruit salad with both your lunch and your supper or choose one of the dessert suggestions given in the recipe section.

- All the recipes serve two unless otherwise stated.

## Day 1

Learn to identify the difference between actual physical hunger and emotional hunger. Before you reach for a chocolate bar or a slice of cake, ask yourself whether you're really hungry. We often turn to food for comfort when we're feeling miserable, stressed, tired, bored or angry. Keeping a food diary (page 108) will help you identify danger times when you're more likely to overeat.

**Breakfast**
Apple and Blackberry Muesli (page 118).

**Lunch**
Stuffed Portobello Mushrooms (page 119).

**Supper**
Roasted Vegetables with Brown Rice (page 133).

## Day 2

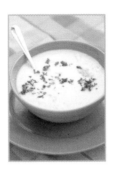

Give food your full attention. Focus on it and eat slowly, making the time to sit down and enjoy your meals at the table rather than eating from a tray balanced on your knees in front of the TV. If you don't concentrate on what you're eating, you are more likely to miss the signals saying you are full. The brain takes fifteen minutes to get the message that the stomach is full, so if you eat too quickly, your stomach fills up before your brain knows it and you will end up eating too much.

**Breakfast**
Stir 1 tbsp apricot conserve, 30g chopped ready to eat apricots and 1 tbsp sugar-free muesli into 150g plain low-fat bio yoghurt.

**Lunch**
Smoked Haddock and Sweetcorn Chowder (page 121).

**Supper**
Chicken Stuffed with Brie on a Bed of Leeks (page 133) and 150g (cooked weight) baby new potatoes.

## Day 3

Learn to have a healthy relationship with food. Don't deny yourself the foods you enjoy or feel bad if you occasionally succumb to temptation, this will simply create negative feelings making your diet more likely to fail in the long run. Instead, learn to eat the foods you really want, but in smaller quantities.

**Breakfast**
One slice of wholemeal toast spread with 2 tsp of peanut butter topped with 1 small mashed banana.

**Lunch**
Watercress Soup (page 119) and a 50g wholemeal roll.

**Supper**
A ready meal to the value of 400 calories.

## Day 4

Shop smart. Picture your new streamlined body as you do your weekly shop and you'll be less tempted to buy those fattening foods you know you won't be able to resist once you get home.

**Breakfast**
One poached egg on one slice of wholemeal toast thinly spread with butter or margarine, 60g poached mushrooms, one grilled tomato.

**Lunch**
Spinach and Feta Frittata (see page 122).

**Supper**
Pizza (page 134).

## Day 5

Change the way you think about food. Studies show that successful dieters are those people who learn how to change both their eating habits and their attitude towards food.

**Breakfast**
One crumpet spread with 2 tsp lemon curd and one low-fat yoghurt

**Lunch**
Devilled Mushrooms (page 123).

**Supper**
Griddled Chicken with Salsa Verde (page 134) and 150g baby new potatoes.

## Day 6

Eat regularly. Eating little and often will help curb hunger pangs, so make sure you have a selection of healthy snacks on hand. Never skip meals, and don't allow yourself to get over-hungry as you'll be more tempted to snack and more likely to overeat at your next meal. Aim to eat three small- to medium-sized meals a day plus two or three small healthy snacks.

**Breakfast**
Mix 30g branflakes or other high-fibre cereal with a small chopped banana, pour over 200ml semi-skimmed milk.

**Lunch**
Ham and Pea Frittata (page 123) and a large green salad.

**Supper**
Prawns with Pak Choi and Rice Noodles (page 135).

## Day 7

Never skip breakfast. After ten to twelve hours without food our energy reserves are low and our bodies need fuel. What you choose to eat (or not to eat) at breakfast can affect your mood, physical and mental performance, weight and health. Studies show that breakfast eaters tend to be slimmer than breakfast skippers because if you miss breakfast you're more likely to snack during the morning and overeat at lunch. Other studies show that breakfast eaters are also less likely to suffer from colds and flu.

**Breakfast**
Apple Porridge (page 118).

**Lunch**
Tuscan Bean Soup (page 122) and a 50g wholemeal roll.

**Supper**
Thai Fishcakes (page 135).

## Day 8

Start your meal with a bowl of soup. Studies have shown that soup, particularly chunky soup, has a satiating effect, and when soup is eaten as the first course of a meal the total number of calories consumed at that meal was reduced by around 20 per cent.

**Breakfast**
As for Day 1.

**Lunch**
Gazpacho (page 126). Two oat cakes and 75g reduced-fat hummus.

**Supper**
Pork with Broccoli and Black Bean Sauce (page 136).

## Day 9

Forget crash or fad diets – they provide a quick fix to a problem that needs a long-term solution, so they don't work. Successful dieters are those who learn how to change both their eating habits and their attitude towards food permanently.

**Breakfast**
As for Day 2.

**Lunch**
Chicken and Cracked Wheat Salad (page 127).

**Supper**
Pasta with Spicy Tomato Sauce (page 137).

## Day 10

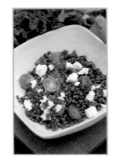

Fill up on high-fibre foods. Wholemeal bread and pasta and wholegrain breakfast cereals are more filling and help you feel full for longer, as well as providing heath benefits.

**Breakfast**
As for Day 3.

**Lunch**
Warm Lentil and Feta Salad (page 124).

**Supper**
Pasta with Peas and Ham (page 137).

## Day 11

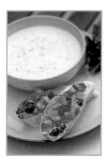

Be realistic. If you set unrealistic goals you're more likely to become disheartened and quit. Aim for a slow but steady weight loss of half a kilo to a kilo a week and you are more likely to keep the weight off.

**Breakfast**
As for Day 4.

**Lunch**
Bowl of vegetable soup and Tomato and Olive Bruschetta (page 129).

**Supper**
Chicken with Lentils (page 138)

## Day 12

Be prepared. Make sure your cupboard is full of healthy foods and you have plenty of low-calorie snacks on hand.

**Breakfast**
As for Day 5.

**Lunch**
Sweet Potato with Cottage Cheese and Crispy Bacon (page 126).

**Supper**
Ready meal to the value of 400 calories.

## Day 13

Avoid all or nothing thinking. Don't feel that one bad day will ruin the whole diet. Life is full of ups and downs – if you've had a bad day be a little stricter with yourself the next.

**Breakfast**
As for Day 6.

**Lunch**
Salad Niçoise (page 127).

**Supper**
Grill 150g cod fillet and serve with a large portion of Ratatouille (page 138) and 150g cooked new potatoes. Serves 1.

## Day 14

Drink at least eight glasses of water a day. It's easy to confuse thirst with hunger, so when you think you're feeling hungry, try drinking a large glass of water first and also drink one before each of your meals.

**Breakfast**
As for Day 7.

**Lunch**
Curried Chicken Salad (page 132).

**Supper**
Stir-fried vegetables, plus 100g prawns.

# Day 15

Chew your food thoroughly. Chewing gets the digestive process off to a good start because it breaks food down into smaller, more manageable pieces, making it easier to swallow. It also mixes food with saliva, which begins the digestion of carbohydrates into simple sugars. Make sure you chew each mouthful carefully before you begin the next.

**Breakfast**
As for Day 2.

**Lunch**
Mushroom and Pasta Salad (page 132).

**Supper**
Tandoori chicken, 100g cooked basmati rice, 3 tbsp tzatziki.

# Day 16

Avoid eating late at night. Studies show that the time of day when you eat your meals has no effect on whether the food is laid down as fat or burnt off as energy, but tucking in to a large meal late at night does increase the risk of heartburn. Aim to eat your evening meal at least two hours before you plan to go to bed to allow plenty of time for your food to digest properly.

**Breakfast**
As for Day 3.

**Lunch**
Cheese salad sandwich: 2 slices of wholemeal bread, 40g grated Cheddar, plenty of salad; or a shop-bought salad to the value of 350 calories.

**Supper**
Fruity Chicken Casserole (page 139) and one medium-sized jacket potato, about 175g.

# Day 17

Avoid drinking tea with meals as the tannin interferes with the absorption of iron from food. Iron deficiency, which results in anaemia, causes tiredness, lack of energy and increased susceptibility to infection, and in a recent survey one in three women in the UK were found to have low iron stores. However, vitamin C increases the absorption of iron from foods, so drink fruit juice or eat fruit and vegetables at the same time as iron-rich foods, such as dark-green leafy vegetables, beans and pulses and wholemeal bread, to boost absorption.

**Breakfast**
As for Day 2.

**Lunch**
Two scrambled eggs on two slices of wholemeal toast.

**Supper**
Beef with Redcurrant Sauce (page 140) and 150g boiled new potatoes.

# Day 18

Taste your food before adding salt. Adding salt is purely a habit – how do you know if you need to add it if you haven't tried the food first? You don't – so taste before you shake! Try using other flavourings such as herbs and spices, lemon juice or mustard rather than salt to flavour your foods.

**Breakfast**
As for Day 4.

**Lunch**
150g baked beans on two slices of wholemeal toast.

**Supper**
Cod Baked with Moroccan Spices (page 140) and 3 tbsp tzatziki.

## Day 19

Avoid temptation. Never go food shopping when you're hungry and always write a list. Don't put serving bowls on the table at meal times. If you know you won't be able to resist second helpings or picking at leftovers, freeze them or throw them away before you sit down to eat.

**Breakfast**
As for Day 5.

**Lunch**
Large bowl of chicken or vegetable soup and a 60g wholemeal roll.

**Supper**
Prawn and Pea Pilaf (page 141).

## Day 20

Don't brush your teeth immediately after eating or drinking acidic foods. The acid in drinks such as fruit juice and in foods such as pickles can weaken the enamel that protects your teeth, making them more susceptible to damage during brushing. Rinse your mouth with a little water after eating acidic foods, but wait for at least 45 minutes before brushing.

**Breakfast**
As for Day 6.

**Lunch**
A ready-prepared salad to the value of 350 calories.

**Supper**
Pork with Mustard and Pasta (page 141).

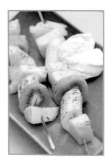

## Day 21

Don't weigh yourself more than once a week. Try to weigh yourself at the same time of day – most people weigh slightly less in the morning than at the end of the day – and always use the same scales and wear the same clothes. Most women will find they gain a little weight in the week before their period. Remember that muscle weighs more than fat, so if you're losing fat but building muscle you may not see any change in your weight.

**Breakfast**
As for Day 7.

**Lunch**
Large bowl of tomato soup and a 60g wholemeal roll.

**Supper**
Vegetable Lasagne (page 142).

## Day 22

Make use of every opportunity to stay active. Instead of using the remote control to change the TV channels, get up. Stand up when you make a telephone call. Use the stairs instead of the lift or escalator; get off the bus one stop early and walk the rest of the way home.

**Breakfast**
As for Day 6.

**Lunch**
Ham salad sandwich: 2 slices of granary or wholemeal bread, a thin scrape of butter or margarine, 60g wafer-thin smoked ham, plenty of salad.

**Supper**
Kedgeree (page 142).

## Day 23

Learn to read food labels. It's worth remembering that 'reduced fat' and 'reduced calorie' doesn't necessarily mean low calorie.

**Breakfast**
As for Day 7.

**Lunch**
60g reduced-fat paté, 75g French bread and 2 tbsp reduced-fat coleslaw.

**Supper**
Lemon Chicken with Egg Fried Rice (page 143).

## Day 24

Say no to nibbles. Nibbles are a dieter's biggest enemy: a handful of peanuts here and a few tortilla chips there may not seem like much, but it all adds up.

**Breakfast**
As for Day 5.

**Lunch**
Sticky Chicken with Sweet and Sour Cucumber (page 130).

**Supper**
Ready meal to the value of 400 calories.

## Day 25

Learn to relax. Don't use overeating as a mechanism for coping with stress.

**Breakfast**
As for Day 4.

**Lunch**
Hummus and carrot sandwich made with 2 slices of wholemeal or granary bread, 75g red-pepper hummus and some grated carrot.

**Supper**
Chicken with Mushroom Stuffing (page 144) and one medium-sized sweet potato, baked.

## Day 26

Eat moderate amounts of fat. Diets that contain between 30-35 per cent of the calories as fat are much more successful in the long term than very low-fat diets.

**Breakfast**
As for Day 3.

**Lunch**
Lentil or vegetable soup and a 60g wholemeal roll.

**Supper**
Plaice with a Roasted Tomato Sauce (page 144).

## Day 27

Adopt a positive outlook and believe you can succeed. Studies show that people who believe they can lose weight are much more successful than those who don't.

**Breakfast**
As for Day 6.

**Lunch**
Brie, watercress and ham sandwich: spread 2 lightly toasted slices of granary bread with a thin layer of reduced-fat mayonnaise, add 50g thinly sliced Brie, 2 slices of wafer-thin ham and plenty of watercress.

**Supper**
Thai Beef Salad (page 145).

## Day 28

Make sure you're eating enough. Eating too few calories forces the body into starvation mode so it holds on to calories, making it more difficult to lose weight.

**Breakfast**
As for Day 1.

**Lunch**
175g baked potato filled with 60g cottage cheese with chives and 60g prawns.

**Supper**
Lemon Crusted Salmon (page 145) and 150g boiled new potatoes.

# Breakfasts

## Apple and Blackberry Muesli

250 calories
1g fat (of which 0.5g saturated fat)
1g fibre

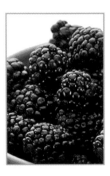

30g sugar-free muesli
150g low-fat bio-yoghurt
1 apple, coarsely grated
50g blackberries or raspberries

Mix the muesli with the yoghurt and stir in the fruit.

## Apple Porridge

300 calories
2g fat (of which 0.5g saturated fat)
1g fibre

30g porridge oats
175ml semi-skimmed milk
1 apple, coarsely grated
1 level tsp sunflower seeds
2 tsp maple syrup

Mix the oats and milk in a saucepan and bring to
the boil. Simmer gently for a couple of minutes. Add
the sunflower seeds and the maple syrup and serve.

# Watercress Soup

200 calories
8g fat (of which 3g saturated fat)
2g fibre

2 tsp groundnut oil
1 onion, finely chopped
125g approx. floury potatoes such as Maris
Piper, peeled and cut into small cubes
1 bunch watercress, washed and drained
    thoroughly and roughly chopped,
    reserving a few whole sprigs for garnish
250ml vegetable or chicken stock
salt and freshly ground black pepper
1 level tbsp cornflour
250ml semi-skimmed milk
2 tbsp half-fat crème fraiche, optional

Heat the oil in a large saucepan. Add the onion
and fry for about 5 minutes, stirring occasionally,
until just beginning to soften. Add the potato and
continue cooking for a further 5 minutes, stirring
occasionally. Add the watercress, stock and
seasoning. Bring to the boil, reduce the heat,
cover and simmer for 15 minutes or until the
potatoes are soft.

Allow to cool slightly, then transfer to a food
processor or blender and process until smooth.

Return the soup to a clean pan. Blend the
cornflour with a little of the milk and stir into the
soup. Add the rest of the milk, bring to the boil
and cook, stirring continuously for 1 minute or until
the soup begins to thicken. Adjust the seasoning.

Serve garnished with crème fraiche and the
reserved watercress.

# Stuffed Portobello Mushrooms

250 calories
6g fat (of which 1g saturated fat)
2g fibre

2 Portobello mushrooms or
    large field mushrooms
1 tbsp olive oil
1 medium-sized red onion, finely chopped
2 sticks celery, finely chopped
75g fresh white breadcrumbs
125g wafer-thin smoked ham, roughly
    chopped
4 tbsp fresh parsley, chopped
zest of 1 large lemon
salt and freshly ground black pepper

Preheat the oven to 220°C/425°F/gas mark 7.

Wipe the mushrooms with a damp cloth.
Remove and finely chop the stalks. Lightly brush
the cap of each mushroom with a little of the
olive oil and place on a baking sheet.

Heat the remaining oil in a frying pan, add the
mushroom stalks, onion and celery and fry over a
medium heat, stirring occasionally, for 3–4 minutes
until the vegetables are beginning to soften. Then
stir in the breadcrumbs, ham, parsley and lemon
zest and season to taste.

Spoon the breadcrumb mixture into the
mushrooms and put into the oven for 15–20
minutes or until the mushrooms are tender.

Serve with a green salad.

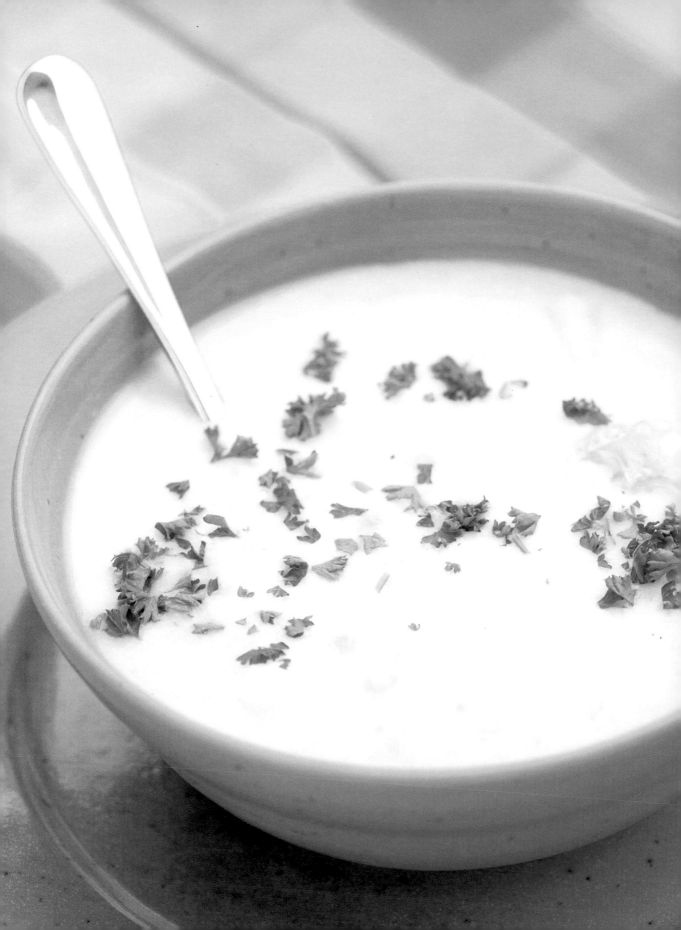

# Smoked Haddock and Sweetcorn Chowder

300 calories
6g fat (of which 1g saturated fat)
4g fibre

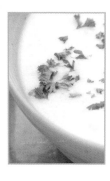

2 tsp groundnut oil
1 medium onion, peeled and finely chopped
250g approx. floury potatoes such as Maris Piper,
   peeled and cut into small cubes
200ml fish stock
150g fresh, frozen or canned sweetcorn,
   thawed and drained if necessary
200ml skimmed milk
200g skinless, smoked haddock fillets,
   cut into bite-sized pieces
salt and freshly ground black pepper
fresh parsley, chopped

Heat the oil in a large saucepan, add the onions and fry over
a gentle heat, stirring occasionally for 5 minutes. Add the
potatoes and continue cooking for a further 2 minutes. Add
the fish stock and bring to the boil. Reduce the heat, cover
and simmer for about 10–15 minutes until the potatoes are
tender. Roughly mash the potatoes into the liquid.

   Add the sweetcorn and the milk and bring back to the boil,
then reduce the heat and simmer for 5 minutes. Stir in the fish
and continue to cook for a further 5 minutes. Season to taste
and garnish with the chopped parsley.

# Tuscan Bean Soup

270 calories
5g fat (of which 1g saturated fat)
15g fibre

2 tsp olive oil
1 small red onion, finely chopped
1 clove garlic, crushed or finely chopped
1 carrot, peeled and diced
2 sticks celery, chopped
400g can chopped tomatoes
1 tbsp sun-dried tomato paste
400ml vegetable stock
2 sprigs fresh thyme
salt and freshly ground black pepper
300g can cooked mixed beans, drained and rinsed
3 tbsp chopped flat-leafed parsley
2 tsp pesto

Heat the oil in a non-stick saucepan and sauté the onion for about 5 minutes or until soft. Stir in the garlic, carrot and celery and continue to cook for a further 5 minutes. Add the tomatoes, tomato paste, stock, thyme and seasoning. Bring to the boil, then reduce the heat to a simmer, cover and simmer, stirring occasionally, for 20–30 minutes or until the vegetables are soft.

Place half the vegetable mixture into a food processor, blend until smooth, then return to the pan. Add the beans, and simmer for a further 10 minutes until they are heated through. Just before serving stir in the chopped parsley.

Garnish with pesto and serve.

# Spinach and Feta Frittata

315 calories
22g fat (of which 8g saturated fat)
2g fibre

200g fresh young spinach, washed
    but not drained
4 eggs, beaten
4 tbsp semi-skimmed milk
salt and freshly ground black pepper
freshly grated nutmeg
2 tsp groundnut oil
50g feta cheese, crumbled

Put the spinach in a large saucepan with just the water that clings to it and simmer for 2–3 minutes or until it is just wilted. Drain well, squeezing out as much liquid as possible, then chop roughly.

Whisk together the eggs, milk, seasoning and nutmeg. Heat the oil in a small non-stick frying pan. Add the spinach and cook over a medium heat, stirring occasionally, for 1–2 minutes. Pour in the beaten egg mixture, sprinkle over the cheese and cook for about 4 minutes or until the bottom of the frittata is just set.

Transfer the frying pan to a pre-heated grill and cook for a further 4–5 minutes or until the frittata is just firm to the touch.

Serve with a tomato salad and crusty wholemeal or granary bread.

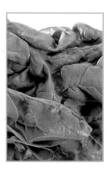

# Devilled Mushrooms

200 calories
5g fat (of which 1g saturated fat)
4g fibre

2 tsp groundnut oil
1 clove garlic, crushed or finely chopped
1 small red onion, chopped
2 tsp soft brown sugar
1 tsp tomato purée
2 tsp Dijon mustard
1 tbsp red wine vinegar
350g chestnut mushrooms, quartered
50ml chicken or vegetable stock
1 tsp Worcestershire sauce
1 tbsp mango chutney
2 slices wholemeal crusty bread, toasted

Heat the oil in a frying pan. Add the garlic and onion and fry, stirring, for 2–3 minutes. Add the sugar, tomato purée and mustard and cook for a further 2 minutes. Add the vinegar and boil until the liquid has almost evaporated.

Add the mushrooms and cook for 5 minutes. Add the stock, Worcestershire sauce and mango chutney, lower the heat and simmer gently for another 10 minutes until the sauce is thick and syrupy.

Spoon the mushrooms on to the toast and serve.

# Ham and Pea Frittata

320 calories
16g fat (of which 5g saturated fat)
2g fibre

4 eggs, beaten
4 tbsp skimmed milk
salt and freshly ground black pepper
2 tsp groundnut oil
3 spring onions, thinly sliced
75g frozen peas, thawed
125g wafer-thin ham, roughly chopped

Whisk together the eggs, milk and seasoning. Heat the oil in a small non-stick frying pan. Add the spring onions and fry for 3–4 minutes until soft. Stir in the peas and the chopped ham.

Pour in the egg mixture and cook for about 4 minutes or until the bottom of the frittata is just set. Transfer the frying pan to a preheated grill and cook for about another 4 minutes until the frittata is just firm to the touch.

# Warm Lentil and Feta Salad

300 calories
9g fat (of which 6g saturated fat)
7g fibre

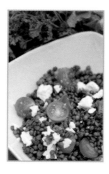

1 × 320g can green lentils, drained and rinsed

300g cherry tomatoes, sliced in half

3 tbsp fresh parsley, chopped

2 tbsp low-fat French dressing

75g feta cheese, crumbled

salt and freshly ground black pepper

Put the lentils in a small pan and gently warm through.
Transfer to a warm serving dish and mix in the tomatoes,
parsley and the dressing. Add the cheese, season to taste
and serve.

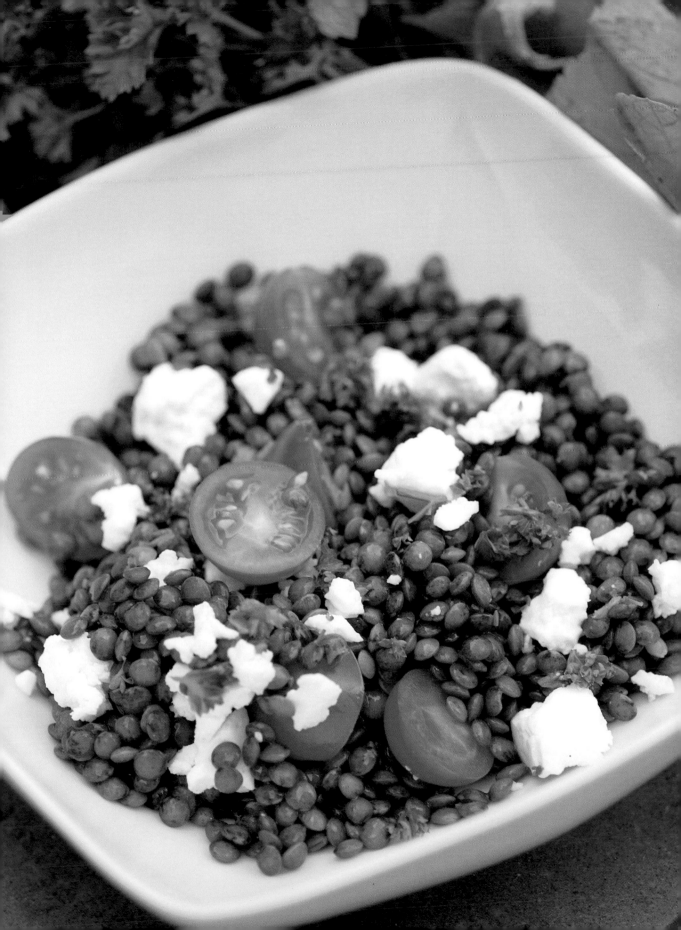

# Sweet Potato with Cottage Cheese and Crispy Bacon

300 calories
6g fat (of which 3g saturated fat)
5g fibre

*Serves 1*
1 medium-sized sweet potato, about 250g
1 rasher lean smoked bacon
100g cottage cheese

Preheat the oven to 200°C/400°F/gas mark 6.

Pierce the potato in several places, wrap it in foil, put it in the oven and bake for 45–60 minutes or until soft.

Cook the bacon under a hot grill until crispy. Roughly chop or crumble it into small pieces. Mix the bacon and the cottage cheese together.

Remove the potato from the foil and slice it in half. Spoon in the bacon and cottage cheese mixture and serve.

# Gazpacho

125 calories
2g fat (of which 1g saturated fat)
4g fibre

½ small red pepper, deseeded and roughly chopped
½ green pepper, deseeded and roughly chopped
½ cucumber, peeled and chopped
1 clove garlic, peeled
¼ small red onion, peeled
3 large ripe plum tomatoes, skin and seeds removed, and roughly chopped
1 tbsp fresh mint, chopped
¼ large red chilli, deseeded and finely chopped
25ml red wine vinegar
15g fresh white breadcrumbs
1 tbsp tomato ketchup
1 tbsp olive oil
½ tsp salt
freshly ground black pepper
425ml cold water

Place all the ingredients in a large bowl. Pour the mixture, in batches, into a food processor or blender and purée until smooth. Check the seasoning and chill for 1–2 hours before serving.

# Chicken and Cracked Wheat Salad

350 calories
13g fat (of which 3g saturated fat)
2g fibre

50g bulgar (cracked) wheat
4 plum tomatoes, deseeded and finely diced
2 spring onions, finely chopped
2 tbps fresh mint, chopped
2 tbsp fresh parsley, chopped
1 tbsp olive oil
juice and zest of ½ a lemon
salt and freshly ground black pepper to taste
2 ready-cooked, skinless chicken breasts,
    sliced into bite-sized pieces

Put the bulgar wheat into a large bowl, cover with plenty of boiling water and leave to stand for 15 minutes. Drain well. Stir in the tomatoes, spring onions, herbs, olive oil, lemon juice and zest and seasoning to taste. Stir in the chicken and serve.

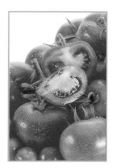

# Salad Niçoise

325 calories
20g fat (of which 3g saturated fat)
4g fibre

*For the dressing*
3 tbsp olive oil
1 tbsp wine vinegar
1 tsp wholegrain mustard
pinch of sugar

*For the salad*
150g French beans, trimmed and sliced in half
125g baby new potatoes, sliced in half
125g cherry tomatoes, sliced in half
50g pitted black olives, roughly chopped
200g can tuna in brine, drained and flaked

To make the dressing whisk together the olive oil, vinegar, mustard and sugar in a jug.

Put the beans in a pan of boiling salted water and cook for about 3 minutes or until just tender. Drain, then plunge them immediately into a bowl of cold water, to prevent them cooking any further, drain again and set aside.

Cook the potatoes in a large pan of salted boiling water until tender. Set aside to cool.

Put the tomatoes, olives, French beans and potatoes in a large bowl and mix well. Stir in the tuna. Drizzle over the dressing and serve immediately.

If you don't have time to make your own dressing use 2 tbsp low-fat French dressing.

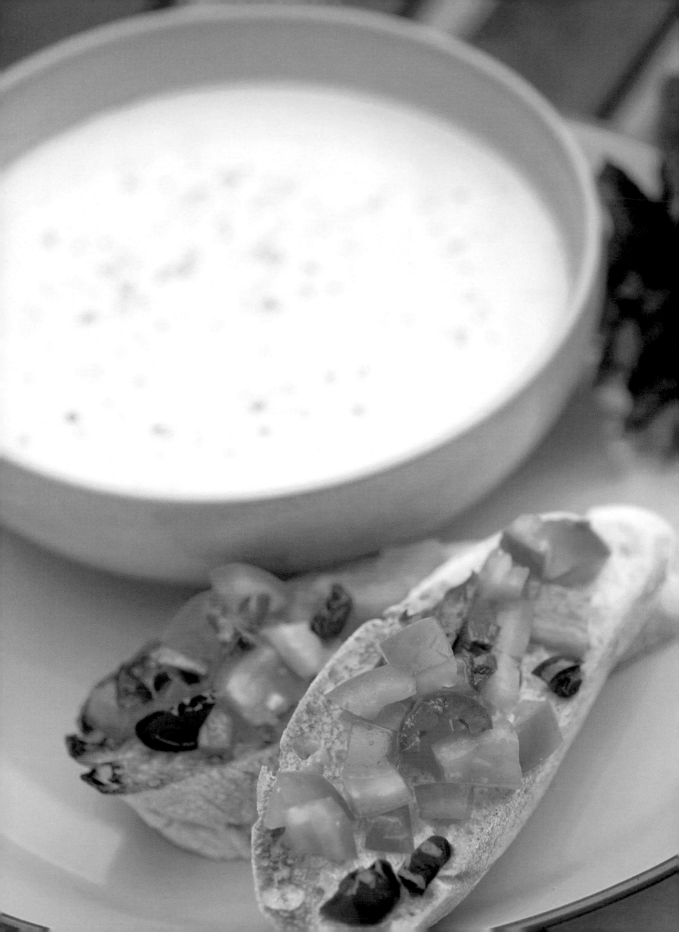

# Tomato and Olive Bruschetta

200 calories
8g fat (of which 2g saturated fat)
3g fibre

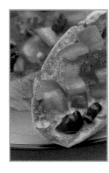

4 ripe plum tomatoes, sliced into quarters and deseeded
25g pitted black olives, roughly chopped
1 tbsp fresh basil, chopped
½ tsp caster sugar
1 tbsp olive oil
salt and freshly ground black pepper
2 × 50g slices bread
1 fat garlic clove
basil leaves to garnish

Mix together the tomatoes, olives, basil, sugar, olive oil
and seasoning. Cover and set aside for 30 minutes.

Put the bread under a preheated grill and toast until
golden brown. Slice the garlic clove in half and rub over
one side of the bread.

Spoon the tomato mixture over the toasted bread.
Garnish with basil and serve.

# Sticky Chicken with Sweet and Sour Cucumber

315 calories

11g fat (of which 3g saturated fat)

2g fibre

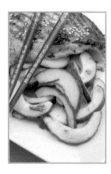

*For the chicken*

4 tbsp mango chutney

2 cloves garlic, crushed or finely chopped

zest of 1 lemon

2 skinless chicken breasts

1 tbsp sesame seeds

*For the cucumber*

½ large cucumber, sliced in half

2 tbsp rice wine vinegar

2 tbsp sweet chilli dipping sauce

2 spring onions, finely chopped

Mix together the mango chutney, garlic and lemon zest. Using a sharp knife make a few deep cuts in the surface of each chicken breast and put it in a shallow dish and spoon over the marinade. Cover and leave the chicken to marinate in the fridge for at least 30 minutes but longer, or overnight, if possible.

Using a small spoon, scoop out and discard the cucumber seeds. Cut the cucumber into 3mm slices and put in a bowl. Add the rice wine vinegar, chilli sauce and spring onions and mix well.

Remove the chicken from the marinade, making sure that the surface of the chicken is well coated with marinade, and put under a hot grill for 5 minutes. Turn the chicken and brush on the remaining marinade. Sprinkle with sesame seeds and continue grilling for a further 5 minutes or until the chicken is cooked through.

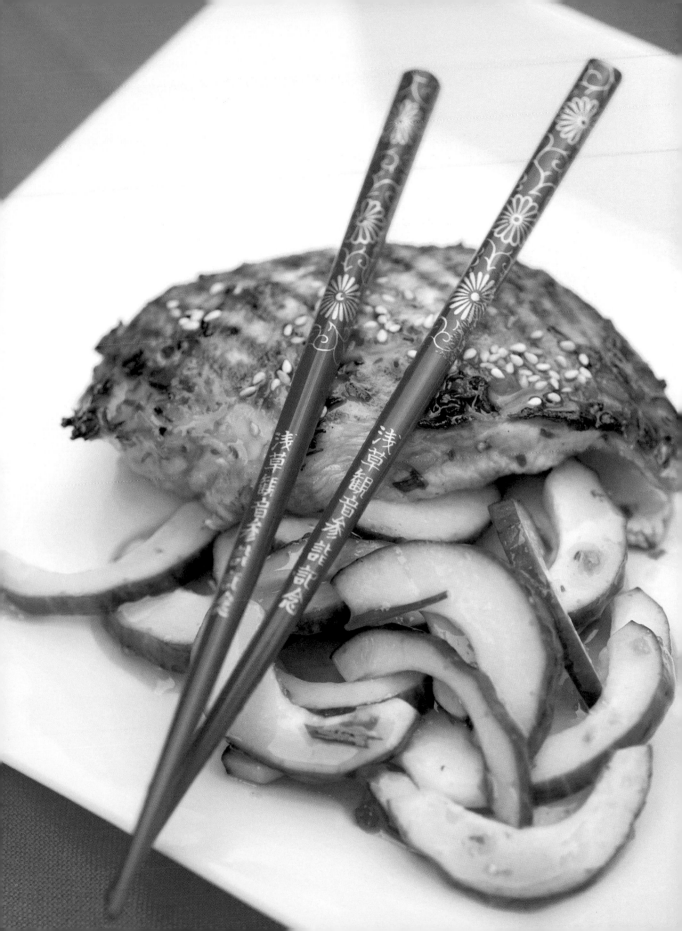

## Mushroom and Pasta Salad

340 calories
11g fat (of which 3g saturated fat)
3g fibre

125g pasta spirals
1 tbsp olive oil
2 spring onions, thinly sliced
150g brown cap mushrooms, roughly chopped
zest and juice of 1 lemon
4 tbsp reduced-fat crème fraiche
salt and freshly ground black pepper

Cook the pasta according to the packet
instructions, then drain, put into a bowl and
allow to cool.

Heat the olive oil in a small frying pan, add
the spring onions and mushrooms and fry for
4–5 minutes. Then add the lemon zest and juice
and continue to cook for a further 3–4 minutes.

Add the mushroom mixture to the pasta,
stir in the crème fraiche and season to taste.

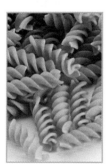

## Curried Chicken Salad

350 calories
11g fat (of which 2g saturated fat)
2g fibre

2 tbsp reduced-fat mayonnaise
2 tbsp natural bio-yoghurt
1 tbsp mango chutney
2 tsp mild curry paste
150g cooked brown rice
2 spring onions, finely chopped
2 sticks celery, finely chopped
4 ready-to-eat dried apricots
200g ready-cooked chicken breasts,
    sliced in to bite sized pieces
salt and freshly ground black pepper

Mix the mayonnaise, yoghurt, mango chutney and
curry paste in a large bowl. Add the rice and mix
well. Stir in the spring onions, celery, apricots and
chicken. Season to taste and serve.

## Roasted Vegetables with Brown Rice

390 calories
14g fat (of which 2g saturated fat)
10g fibre

1 red and 1 orange pepper, deseeded and cut
   into bite-sized pieces
1 aubergine, cut into bite-sized pieces
3 thin courgettes, trimmed and cut into
   bite-sized pieces
2 small red onions, peeled and cut into quarters
1 bulb fennel, trimmed and thickly sliced
4 cloves garlic
2 tbsp olive oil
salt and freshly ground black pepper
8 cherry tomatoes

Preheat the oven to 220°C/425°F/gas mark 7.
   Put the peppers, aubergine, courgettes, onions,
fennel and garlic in a large roasting tin. Drizzle over
the oil and mix well to ensure that all the vegetables
become coated in oil. Season to taste and put in
the oven for 20 minutes. Add the tomatoes and
cook for a further 5 minutes or until all the
vegetables are tender.
   Serve with a 100g of cooked brown rice
per serving.

## Chicken Stuffed with Brie on a Bed of Leeks

380 calories
21g fat (of which 11g saturated fat)
2g fibre

2 skinless chicken breasts
75g Brie
4 slices Parma ham
2 tsp butter
2 large leeks, washed, drained and
   thinly sliced
50ml chicken stock
salt and freshly ground black pepper

Preheat the oven to 190°C/375°F/gas mark 5.
   With a sharp knife make a lengthways cut
through each chicken breast to create a pocket.
Cut the cheese into two pieces and stuff one in
each pocket. Wrap 2 slices of Parma ham round
each breast, and secure them with a cocktail stick.
   Put the chicken on a lightly oiled baking tray and
cook for 35 minutes or until it is cooked through.
   Meanwhile, heat the butter in a large non-stick
frying pan, add the leeks and sauté, tossing from
time to time, for 2–3 minutes. Add the chicken
stock and season. Cover the pan, and continue
cooking for a further 2–3 minutes or until the leeks
are tender.
   Transfer the chicken to a warm plate and serve
with the leeks and their stock.

# Pizza

400 calories
15g fat (of which 7g saturated fat)
2g fibre

### For the pizza

1 × 23cm ready-made thin and crispy pizza base
200g tomato salsa
60g wafer-thin smoked ham
60g reduced-fat mozzarella cheese grated
fresh or dried herbs

### For the tomato salsa

4 plum tomatoes
½ red onion, finely chopped
salt and freshly ground black pepper
1 tbsp olive oil

Preheat the oven to 220°C/425°F/gas mark 7.

Cover 4 plum tomatoes with boiling water and allow to stand for 1 minute. Drain the tomatoes and plunge into a bowl of ice-cold water. Peel the tomatoes, remove the seeds and dice the flesh. Mix with ½ finely chopped red onion, seasoning to taste and 1 tbsp of olive oil.

Spread the pizza base with the rest of the ingredients and bake for 15–20 minutes. Serve with a large green salad with low-fat dressing.

# Griddled Chicken with Salsa Verde

380 calories
28g fat (of which 5g saturated fat)
0g fibre

### For the salsa verde

2 tsp capers
1 garlic clove, peeled and roughly chopped
2 tsp Dijon mustard
4 tbsp flat-leafed parsley
4 tbsp fresh mint
2 anchovy fillets
juice and zest of 1 lemon
4 tbsp olive oil

### For the chicken

2 skinless chicken breasts,
    sliced almost in half lengthways
1 tsp olive oil
salt and freshly ground black pepper

To make the salsa verde, put all the ingredients in a food processor or blender and process until smooth.

Lay the chicken between sheets of greaseproof paper and beat them with a rolling pin until about 5mm thick. Brush each side of the chicken with the olive oil.

Heat a griddle pan until hot and cook the chicken for 4–5 minutes on each side until cooked through.

Transfer to a plate, drizzle over the salsa verde and serve.

# Prawns with Pak Choi and Rice Noodles

360 calories
8g fat (of which 1g saturated fat)
4g fibre

100g dried rice noodles
1 tbsp groundnut oil
1 small onion, finely chopped
1 clove garlic, thinly sliced
1 red chilli, deseeded and finely chopped
2.5 cm piece fresh root ginger,
   peeled and finely chopped
1 tbsp light soy sauce
1 tbsp Thai fish sauce
juice of 1 lime
175g mangetout
75g beansprouts
1 small head of pak choi or Chinese cabbage,
washed, drained and trimmed
150g cooked and peeled tiger prawns
small handful fresh coriander, chopped
lime wedges

Prepare the rice noodles according to the packet instructions. Drain and rinse well.

Heat the oil in a large wok or frying pan. Add the onion, garlic, chilli and ginger and stir-fry for 2 minutes. Add the noodles, soy sauce, fish sauce and lime juice, mix well and stir-fry for another 2 minutes. Add the mangetout, beansprouts, pak choi and prawns and continue stir-frying for 2–3 minutes or until the vegetables are cooked.

Garnish with chopped fresh coriander and lime wedges.

# Thai Fish Cakes

215 calories
7g fat (of which 1g saturated fat)
0g fibre

400g skinless cod or haddock fillets
4 spring onions, finely chopped
1 red chilli, deseeded and finely chopped
15ml Thai fish sauce
15ml lime juice
pinch salt
3 tbsp fresh coriander, chopped
1 tbsp sesame oil
lime wedges

Put the first 6 ingredients in a food processor and blend until smooth. Stir in the coriander.

Divide the mixture into 8 and shape it into fish cakes. Put the fish cakes on a plate, cover and chill for an hour to allow them to firm up.

Heat the oil in a shallow frying pan and cook the fish cakes in two batches. Fry them for about 5 minutes on one side then turn and fry for further 3 minutes until they are golden brown.

Serve immediately with wedges of lime to garnish and with stir-fried vegetables.

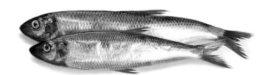

# Pork with Broccoli and Black Bean Sauce

450 calories
17g fat (of which 4g saturated fat)
4g fibre

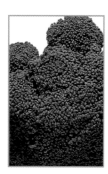

2 tsp vegetable oil

200g pork tenderloin, thinly sliced

1 clove garlic, crushed or finely chopped

2.5cm fresh ginger, finely chopped

4 spring onions, cut into slices 5mm long

75g shiitake mushrooms

100g broccoli, divided into florets

75g baby sweetcorn, sliced lengthways

5 tbsp black bean sauce

2 tsp runny honey

100g egg noodles

1 tsp sesame oil

spring onions, thinly sliced, to garnish

Heat 1 tsp of the oil in a wok or a large frying pan, add the pork and stir-fry over a high heat for 5 minutes or until browned. Remove from the pan and set aside.

Wipe the wok clean with kitchen paper and add the remaining vegetable oil. Once the oil is hot, add the garlic, ginger and spring onions and stir-fry for 1 minute. Add the mushrooms, broccoli and sweetcorn and continue cooking for 2–3 minutes. Return the pork to the pan, stir in the black bean sauce, honey and 100ml water and simmer for a further 5 minutes or until the sauce is hot.

Cook the noodles according to the packet instructions. Drain well then stir through the sesame oil.

To serve, put the noodles and pork in a bowl and garnish with the spring onions.

# Pasta with Spicy Tomato Sauce

435 calories
12g fat (of which 4g saturated fat)
4g fibre

2 tsp olive oil
1 red onion, finely chopped
1 clove garlic, crushed or finely chopped
large pinch of chilli flakes
1 level tsp ground cumin
1 level tsp ground coriander
400g tin chopped tomatoes
1 tbsp tomato purée
100ml red wine
salt and freshly ground black pepper
125g pasta
100g ricotta cheese
handful fresh basil, chopped

Heat the oil in a large saucepan, add the onion,
garlic, chilli, cumin and coriander and fry for
5 minutes until the onions are beginning to soften.
Add the tomatoes, tomato purée and red wine and
season to taste. Bring to the boil, then lower the
heat and simmer gently for about 30 minutes or
until the sauce is reduced by half.

Cook the pasta according to the packet
instructions and drain well.

Transfer the pasta to a serving dish, spoon over
the tomato sauce then top with the ricotta cheese.
Garnish with the fresh basil and serve immediately.

# Pasta with Peas and Ham

450 calories
18g fat (of which 8g saturated fat)
4g fibre

100g penne or a pasta of your choice
90g frozen peas
100g reduced-fat crème fraiche
2 tbsp wholegrain mustard
150g wafer-thin smoked ham, roughly chopped
salt and freshly ground black pepper

Cook the pasta according to packet instructions.
About 3–4 minutes before it has finished cooking
add the peas to the saucepan and continue to cook.
Drain well and return to the pan. Stir in the rest of
the ingredients and season to taste.

## Ratatouille

150 calories
5g fat (of which 1g saturated fat)
8g fibre

2 tsp olive oil
1 red onion, sliced
1 clove garlic, chopped
2 courgettes, sliced
I red pepper, diced
1 aubergine, diced
400g tin chopped tomatoes
1 tbsp tomato purée
salt and freshly ground black pepper

Heat the olive oil in a large non-stick saucepan.
Add the onion and garlic and cook for 3–4 minutes.
Add the courgettes, red pepper, aubergine,
tomatoes, tomato purée and salt and pepper to
taste. Bring to the boil then reduce the heat and
simmer for 20 minutes.

## Chicken with Lentils

400 calories
9g fat (of which 2g saturated fat)
6g fibre

2 tsp olive oil plus a little more
1 small onion, chopped
1 clove garlic, crushed
3 sticks celery, finely chopped
320g canned green lentils
salt and freshly ground black pepper
2 skinless chicken breasts

Heat the oil in a frying pan. Add the onion, garlic
and celery and cook for 5 minutes. Add the lentils
and season to taste. Cook for a further 5 minutes
or until the lentils are hot.

Slice the chicken breasts almost in half
lengthways and lay them between 2 sheets of
greaseproof paper and beat them with a rolling pin
until they're about 5mm thick. Brush each side of
the chicken with olive oil. Heat a griddle pan until
hot then add the chicken and cook for 4–5 minutes
on each side until cooked thoroughly.

Serve with the lentil mixture.

# Fruity Chicken Casserole

500 calories
13g fat (of which 3g saturated fat)
8g fibre

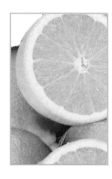

1 clove garlic, crushed or finely chopped
1 tsp fresh ginger, finely chopped
1 red chilli, deseeded and finely chopped
1 cinnamon stick
5 tbsp orange juice
2 skinless chicken breasts, cut into 5cm cubes
2 tsp vegetable oil
6 shallots, peeled
2 tsp plain flour
1 tbsp tomato purée
100ml chicken stock
5 tbsp sherry
salt and freshly ground black pepper
50g ready-to-eat dried apricots
300g tin cooked chickpeas, drained and rinsed
handful fresh coriander, chopped

Place the garlic, ginger, chilli, cinnamon stick and orange
juice in a large bowl. Add the chicken. Cover and leave in
a cool place for at least an hour and preferably overnight.

Preheat the oven to 180°C/350°F/gas mark 4.

Heat the oil in a large flameproof casserole. Remove the
chicken from the marinade and fry over a high heat until lightly
browned, then remove with a slotted spoon and set aside.
Reduce the heat and add a little more oil if necessary. Cook the
shallots for 3 minutes or until just beginning to brown. Return the
chicken to the casserole and stir in the flour and tomato purée
and continue cooking for a further minute, stirring continually.

Add the reserved marinade, stock and sherry and season.
Bring to the boil, then cover and put in the oven for an hour.
Add the apricots and chickpeas and return to the oven for
a further 15 minutes.

Garnish with the fresh coriander and serve with
steamed broccoli.

# Beef with Redcurrant Sauce

280 calories
8g fat (of which 2g saturated fat)
1g fibre

*For the sauce*
2 tsp olive oil
1 small red onion, finely chopped
1 clove garlic, crushed or finely chopped
250ml chicken stock
250ml red wine
½ tsp fresh thyme, chopped
2 level tsp Dijon mustard
salt and freshly ground black pepper
1 level tbsp redcurrant jelly

a little olive oil
2 × 100g rump steak

Heat the oil in a non-stick frying pan, add the onion and garlic and fry, stirring occasionally, for about 5 minutes. Add the stock, red wine, thyme and mustard and bring to the boil. Allow the sauce to bubble for about 10 minutes or until the liquid is thick and syrupy and has reduced by half. Strain the sauce and discard the onions. Season to taste and stir in the redcurrant jelly.

Brush a heavy-based frying pan or griddle with a little olive oil. Heat the pan until very hot, then add the steak and cook to your preference. For cooking times see Cook's Tip on page 145.

Transfer to a warmed serving plate, spoon over a little of the sauce and serve with green vegetables.

# Cod Baked with Moroccan Spices

165 calories
6g fat (of which 1g saturated fat)
0g fibre

2 cloves garlic, crushed or finely chopped
½ tsp ground cumin
½ tsp ground turmeric
¼ tsp paprika
¼ tsp hot chilli powder
zest and juice of 1 lemon
1 tbsp olive oil
1 tbsp fresh parsley, chopped
1 tbsp fresh coriander, chopped
2 × 150g cod fillet

Combine the garlic, spices, lemon zest and juice, olive oil and herbs. Put the fish on a lightly oiled baking tray and put a thick coating of the spice mixture on each piece of fish. Cover loosely with plastic wrap, transfer to the fridge and allow to marinate for an hour.

Preheat the oven to 180°C/350°F/gas mark 4 and bake the fish for 15 minutes or until it turns opaque.

Serve with French beans and tzatziki.

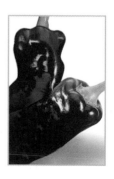

# Prawn and Pea Pilaf

450 calories
8g fat (of which 1g saturated fat)
6g fibre

2 tsp olive oil
1 onion, finely chopped
150g button mushrooms, cut into quarters
½ level tsp ground cumin
½ level tsp cayenne pepper
1 level tbsp tomato purée
125g long grain brown rice
200g tin chopped tomatoes
125g frozen peas
400ml chicken or vegetable stock
salt and freshly ground black pepper
200g cooked and peeled king prawns
juice and zest of 1 lemon
fresh parsley, chopped
lemon wedges

Heat the oil in a large frying pan. Add the onion and mushrooms and fry over a medium heat for about 5 minutes. Stir in the spices and tomato purée and continue to fry for 2–3minutes, stirring frequently. Add the rice and cook the mixture for a further 5 minutes or until the rice starts to turn opaque. Stir continuously. Then add the tomatoes, peas, stock and seasoning and simmer, stirring occasionally, for 35–40 minutes until the rice is tender.

Add the prawns, lemon juice and zest and continue cooking for a further 2–3 minutes until the prawns are heated through.

Serve garnished with a little chopped parsley and lemon wedges.

# Pork with Mustard and Pasta

500 calories
19g fat (of which 6g saturated fat)
4g fibre

125g dried pasta shapes
1 tbsp olive oil
200g lean pork fillet, trimmed of fat
  and cut into thin strips
2 cloves garlic, crushed or finely chopped
125g button mushrooms, roughly chopped
1 bunch of baby leeks, washed and thinly sliced
5 tbsp dry cider or apple juice
3 tbsp wholegrain mustard
salt and freshly ground black pepper
4 tbsp half-fat crème fraiche
fresh chives, chopped

Cook the pasta in plenty of boiling water until just tender. Once the pasta is cooked, drain well.

Heat half the oil in a large non-stick frying pan. Add the pork and fry over a high heat for 4–5 minutes until well browned. Remove the pork with a slotted spoon and set aside.

Reduce the heat slightly and add the remaining oil, the garlic, mushrooms and leeks. Fry over a medium heat for 3–5minutes, stirring occasionally. Add the cider or apple juice and simmer until mushrooms are done, about 5 minutes. Stir in the pork, pasta, mustard and a little salt and black pepper and continue to cook until piping hot.

Add the crème fraiche and serve immediately garnished with chopped chives.

# Vegetable Lasagne

500 calories
25g fat (of which 12g saturated fat)
5g fibre

2 cloves garlic
1 courgette, roughly chopped
1 red pepper, deseeded and chopped
1 red onion, roughly chopped
1 small aubergine, roughly chopped
1 tbsp olive oil
salt and freshly ground black pepper
100g ricotta cheese
1 egg, beaten
4 tbsp skimmed milk
4 tbsp Parmesan cheese, freshly grated
400g ready-made arrabiata sauce
4–6 sheets fresh lasagne,
    or of the dried pre-cooked type

Preheat the oven to 190°C/375°F/gas mark 5.
    Put the garlic and all the chopped vegetables in a large shallow roasting tin. Pour over the oil, season well and toss everything so the vegetables are thoroughly coated with oil. Roast for 30–40 minutes until just tender. Leave to cool slightly.
    Meanwhile, mix together the ricotta, the egg, milk and 2 tbsp of the Parmesan. Season well and set aside.
    Spoon the roasted vegetables into a large bowl and mix with the arrabiata sauce. Spoon half the vegetable and tomato mixture over the base of a lightly greased ovenproof dish. Cover with a layer of lasagne sheets. Add the remaining vegetable mixture and a final layer of pasta. Spread the cheese mixture evenly over the top of the lasagne and sprinkle over the remaining Parmesan. Bake for 30 minutes or until golden brown and bubbling.
    Leave to stand for 5 minutes before serving. Serve with a tomato and basil salad.

# Kedgeree

400 calories
9g fat (of which 1.5g saturated fat)
0.5g fibre

200g undyed smoked haddock fillet
50ml skimmed milk
1 bay leaf
6 peppercorns
100g basmati rice
2 tsp olive oil
4 spring onions, chopped
2 tsp mild curry paste
1 tbsp lemon juice
2 tbsp fresh parsley, chopped
salt and freshly ground black pepper
1 egg, hard boiled, shelled and cut into quarters
fresh parsley, chopped
lemon wedges

Put the fish in a shallow pan. Pour over the milk and add the bay leaf and peppercorns. Cover and simmer gently for about 10 minutes until tender. Drain. Using two forks separate the fish into flakes removing any skin and bones.
    Cook the rice in plenty of boiling, salted water for about 12 minutes. Drain and rinse with hot water to separate the grains.
    Heat the oil in a large non-stick frying pan and stir-fry the spring onions for 1–2 minutes until softened. Stir in the curry paste and cook for a further minute. Add the rice and the fish and keep stirring until it is hot. Add the parsley and lemon juice and season to taste.
    Turn the kedgeree on to a warm serving dish and garnish with the egg, more parsley and lemon wedges.

# Lemon Chicken with Egg Fried Rice

500 calories
15g fat (of which 3g saturated fat)
4g fibre

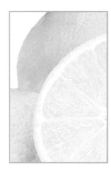

*For the Lemon Chicken*

juice of ½ lemon

1 tbsp dark soy sauce

2 tbsp sweet chilli sauce

1 tsp runny honey

2 tsp groundnut oil

2 skinless chicken breasts, cut into thin strips

2.5 cm piece fresh root ginger, peeled and
   finely chopped

1 red chilli, deseeded and finely chopped

2 cloves garlic, crushed or finely chopped

200g sugar snap peas, trimmed

150g broccoli, divided into small florets

1 tsp sesame seeds

*For the rice*

2 tsp sesame oil

4 spring onions

½ red pepper, diced

100g cooked basmati rice

1 large egg, beaten

Mix the lemon juice, soy sauce, sweet chilli sauce and
honey together in a small bowl.

Heat 1 tsp of the groundnut oil in a large non-stick wok
or frying pan. Add the chicken and stir-fry over a high heat
for 4–5 minutes until cooked through. Remove from the pan
and set aside. Add the remaining groundnut oil to the pan,
reduce the heat, then add the ginger, chilli and garlic and
stir-fry for a 1–2 minutes. Add the vegetables and the
sesame seeds and pour in the sauce, together with 2 tbsp
of water. Cover and simmer for 2–3 minutes. Return the
chicken to the pan and simmer for a further 1–2 minutes.

Heat the sesame oil in another wok or frying pan,
add the spring onions and red pepper and cook for
3–4 minutes. Then add the rice and egg and stir-fry over a
moderate heat for about 5 minutes or until heated through.

Serve immediately in bowls.

## Chicken with Mushroom Stuffing

350 calories
16g fat (of which 10g saturated fat)
0.5g fibre

10g dried mushrooms, well washed
15g butter
75g brown cap mushrooms, chopped
75g low-fat cream cheese
salt and freshly ground black pepper
2 skinless chicken breasts
4 slices Parma ham

Preheat the oven to 190°C/375°F/gas mark 5.

Pour 150ml boiling water over the dried mushrooms and leave them to stand for 15 minutes. Drain and finely chop.

Heat the butter in a large frying pan, add the fresh and dried mushrooms and fry over a medium heat for 10 minutes or until they are beginning to brown and any liquid has evaporated. Remove from the pan and allow to cool.

Put the cream cheese in a bowl, stir in the mushrooms and season to taste.

Using a sharp knife make a lengthways slit in each chicken breast. Spoon in the mushroom mixture. Wrap 2 slices of ham round each chicken breast and enclose in a loose foil parcel. Bake in the oven for 30 minutes until the chicken is cooked.

Remove the chicken from the foil and slice. Serve with sugar snap peas.

## Plaice with a Roasted Tomato Sauce

325 calories
10g fat (of which 3g saturated fat)
4g fibre

1 small red pepper, deseeded
   and roughly chopped
4 plum tomatoes, skinned and roughly chopped
2 sticks celery, roughly chopped
2 cloves garlic
1 tbsp olive oil
salt and freshly ground black pepper
2 large plaice fillets
2 level tbsp pesto
5 tbsp dry white wine

Preheat the oven to 220°C/425°F/gas mark 7.

Put the pepper, tomatoes, celery and garlic in a large roasting tin, drizzle over the olive oil and season with salt and pepper. Cook for 15–20 minutes until the vegetables are soft.

Meanwhile, remove the skin from the plaice fillets (if you buy the fish from a fishmonger they will do this for you). Lay the fish skin-side up on a board and spread 1 tbsp of the pesto over each fillet. Roll the fish up as you would a Swiss roll.

Pour the wine into a flameproof casserole and put the fish in with the seam side of the roll facing down. Bring the wine to the boil. Cover the casserole with a lid or foil, reduce the heat and simmer for about 10 minutes. Using a slotted spoon remove the fish and place on a warm serving dish. Reserve the wine.

Liquidize the roasted vegetables and the wine in food processor or liquidizer for 2–3 minutes until you have a smooth sauce. Pour the sauce back into the casserole, reheat and season to taste.

Serve to accompany the fish.

# Thai Beef Salad

325 calories
10g fat (of which 3g saturated fat)
4g fibre

150g rump or sirloin steak
75g baby sweetcorn
½ large cucumber, sliced in half lengthways
½ small red onion, peeled and finely chopped
2 tbsp fresh coriander, chopped
2 tbsp rice wine vinegar
2 tbsp sweet chilli dipping sauce
1 tbsp sesame seeds, lightly toasted
1 spring onion, thinly sliced

Put the steak on a hot griddle pan and cook until medium rare (see Cook's Tip). Allow it to rest for 10–15 minutes, then slice thinly.

Cook the sweetcorn in a pan of boiling water for 3–4 minutes until tender. Refresh under cold water and drain well.

Using a small spoon scoop out and discard the seeds of the cucumber and cut it into 3mm slices.

Put the beef, sweetcorn, red onions, cucumber and coriander in a large bowl. Stir in the rice wine vinegar and chilli sauce and mix well.

Toast the sesame seeds in a dry frying pan until they begin to brown then garnish the steak with the sesame seeds and the spring onions.

## Cook's Tip

As a rough guide, a 2cm-thick steak should be grilled for about 2 minutes on either side for rare, 3–4 minutes each side for medium, 6–7minutes for well done.

# Lemon Crusted Salmon

335 calories
20g fat (of which 5g saturated fat)
0.5g fibre

3 slices white bread, crusts removed
4 tbsp flat-leafed parsley, chopped
zest of 1 large lemon
10g butter
salt and freshly ground black pepper
2 × 125g salmon cutlets

Place the bread, parsley, lemon zest, butter and seasoning in a food processor and process until you have fine crumbs.

Put the salmon under a moderately hot grill and cook for 5 minutes. Turn it over and top with the breadcrumb mixture, pressing it down gently with the palm of your hand. Cook for a further 5 minutes or until the salmon is cooked through.

Serve with French beans.

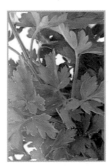

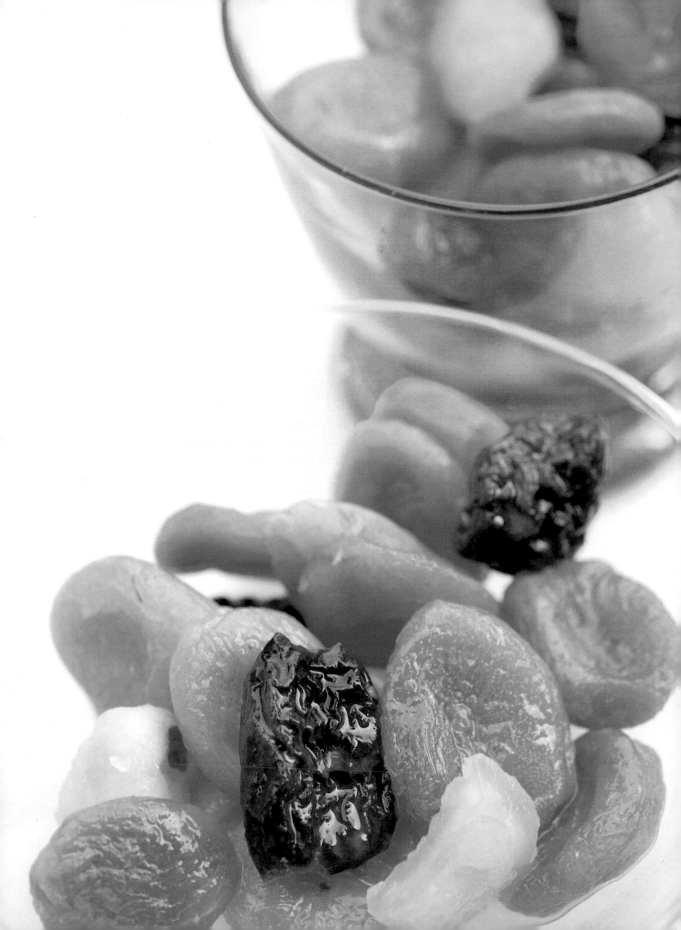

# Spiced Fruit Compote

120 calories
0.5g fat (of which 0g saturated fat)
4g fibre

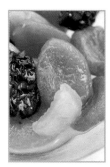

125g mixed dried fruits of your choice
1 cinnamon stick
2 whole green cardamom pods, lightly crushed
200ml apple and mango juice
2 level tsp arrowroot

Put the dried fruit, cinnamon and cardamom in a large bowl. Pour over the juice and 200ml of boiling water. Allow to cool, cover, and leave overnight in the fridge.

Remove the cardamom and cinnamon. Mix the arrowroot with enough cold water to make a smooth paste. Drain the liquid from the fruit into a small saucepan, stir in the arrowroot and bring to boil, cooking for 1 minute or until thickened.

# Banana Parcels

185 calories
9g fat (of which 6g saturated fat)
1g fibre

2 small ripe bananas, thickly sliced
1 tbsp demerera sugar
20g butter
zest of 1 lemon
2 sheets filo pastry, 40 cm × 28.5 cm
maple syrup
a few pistachio nuts, chopped

Preheat the oven to 200°C/400°F/gas mark 6.

Put the bananas in a bowl and sprinkle over the sugar. Melt half the butter in a small pan, add the banana mixture and cook over a low heat for 10 minutes. Remove from the heat, stir in the lemon zest. Allow to cool, then chill in the fridge.

Melt the remaining butter in a small clean pan. Lay one sheet of filo pastry on the work surface, and brush it lightly with melted butter. Fold into three lengthways. Spoon a quarter of the banana mixture on to the pastry about 4 cm from one end. Fold the left corner of the filo diagonally across to the right side of the pastry to cover the filling. Continue folding in the same way until you reach the end of the sheet. Repeat with the remaining sheets of filo and banana.

Place the turnovers on a lightly greased baking sheet, brush with a little more melted butter and bake for 15 minutes or until golden. Drizzle over a little maple syrup and sprinkle with a few chopped pistachio nuts before serving.

Serve with frozen yoghurt or low-fat Greek yoghurt.

# Banana Ice

180 calories
4g fat (of which 3g saturated fat)
1g fibre

2 large bananas, peeled and thickly sliced
150ml semi-skimmed milk
2 tsp maple syrup or honey
1 small chocolate flake, crumbled

Put the bananas in a freezer-proof container and freeze for about 3 hours or until frozen solid. Place the frozen bananas, milk and maple syrup or honey in a blender and process until smooth.

Divide the mixture between two dishes. Sprinkle half the chocolate over each dish and serve immediately.

## Fresh Dates Stuffed with Low-fat Soft Cheese

150 calories
6g fat
1g fibre

75g low-fat soft cheese
1 tbsp icing sugar
zest of 1 orange
6 fresh dates, stoned
sliced orange

Mix together the cheese, icing sugar and orange zest. Stuff each date with a little of this mixture and serve with slices of orange.

## Spiced Plums

80 calories
0g fat
2g fibre

300g ripe plums, stoned and quartered
1 tbsp caster sugar
pinch of ground cinnamon

Put the plums in a small pan with the sugar, cinnamon and 1 tbsp water. Simmer over a gentle heat, stirring occasionally, for 8–10 minutes or until they are soft.

## Baked Pears with a Marmalade Sauce

100 calories
0g fat
1g fibre

*For the pears*
2 ripe pears, peeled, halved and cored
1 tbsp demerera sugar
6 tbsp orange juice

*For the marmalade sauce*
300ml orange juice, less 6 tbsp
1 tbsp orange marmalade
2 tsp arrowroot

Preheat the oven to 200°C/400°F/gas mark 6.

Put each pear on a large square of foil and draw the edges together to make a parcel. Before you close the parcel completely, add 1 tbsp demerera sugar and 3 tbsp of orange juice to each one. Bake for 20 minutes until soft.

To make the sauce, place the remaining orange juice in a small saucepan and stir in the marmalade. Mix the arrowroot with enough water to make a paste and stir into the orange juice. Bring the sauce to the boil and allow to bubble for 1–2 minutes or until it begins to thicken.

Pour over the pears and serve.

# Grilled Fruit Skewers with Lime and Ginger Syrup

80 calories
0g fat
1g fibre

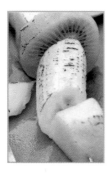

*For the fruit skewer*
1 kiwi fruit, peeled and thickly sliced
2 thick slices of fresh pineapple, cut into quarters
1 small banana, thickly sliced
1 small mango, peeled and cut into thick slices
1 tsp butter, melted

*For the syrup*
juice and zest of 1 lime
1 tbsp chopped crystallized ginger
2 tbsp syrup from the jar of ginger

Thread the fruit on to two wooden skewers. Brush with the melted butter and place under a hot grill for 5 minutes, turning occasionally.

To make the sauce, mix the lime juice and zest, crystallized ginger and syrup together.

Drizzle the sauce over the fruit before serving.

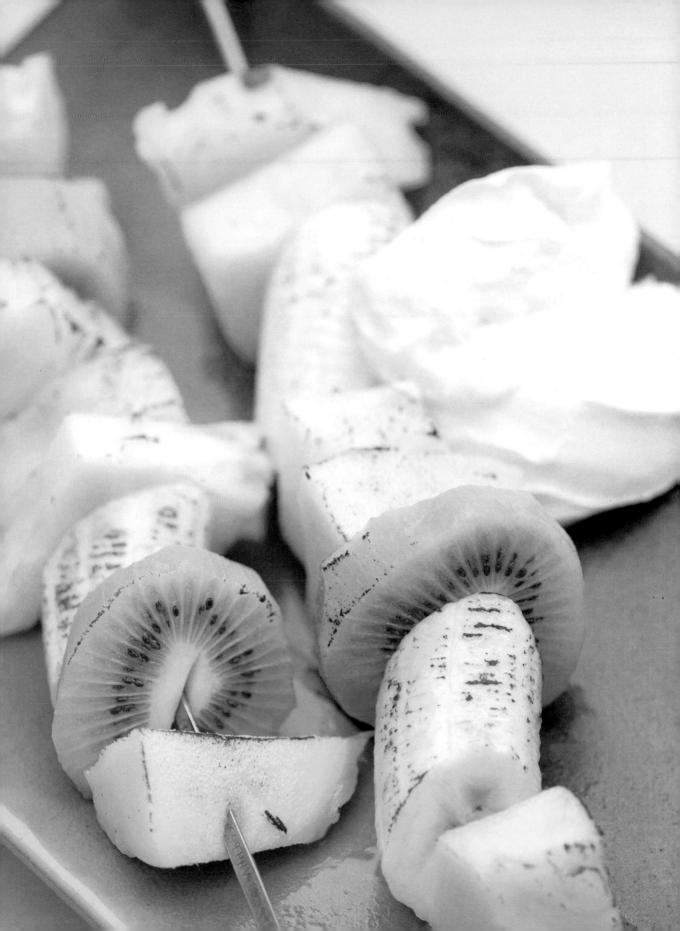

# Keep It Up

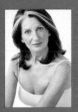

You have finished your 28-day programme and you are thrilled with your new body and you can both feel and see a difference. What next?

Having laid the foundations for vital health and a fantastic body, you will hopefully want to continue with your new way of eating and working out. Keeping yourself motivated is not always easy; you can get stuck in a rut with both your diet and your fitness regime. So try something new. There are many more exercises that you could add to your Pilates workout – look out for other books in the Body Control Pilates range or perhaps try a video (see page 2). We now have a network of Body Control Pilates teachers throughout the country who hold group classes and individual training sessions. If you are lucky enough to live close to a Pilates studio then you might like to try a workout using the studio machinery. You can find information on qualified teachers and Pilates studios on page 2.

It makes good sense to try different aerobic activities because this challenges new muscle groups and new co-ordination skills. If you have been attending aerobic classes try a dance class as well, if you love power walking, add hill walking (press the incline button on the treadmill!). Fitness clubs are constantly adding new classes to their timetables and now you have a new, stronger body be bold and adventurous.

While good health and fitness is a noble goal it should never become an obsession; it is a means to an end, rather than an end in itself. Ask yourself why you want to be healthier, fitter and slimmer? Hopefully you will answer 'so that I can enjoy life more'. This was exactly what Joseph Pilates believed. He thought that the pursuit of health and fitness was not just a physical and emotional responsibility but a moral one as well. He believed we have to take responsibility for our own wellbeing, and be disciplined enough to practise the exercises faithfully. He lived by the dictum 'a sound mind in a sound body'. In his book *Return to Life* the expresses concern about the stresses of modern life: working in offices, pollution in cities, the lack of social or relaxation time. He advocated, 'The attainment and maintenance of a uniformly developed body with a sound mind fully capable of naturally, easily and satisfactorily performing our many and varied daily tasks with spontaneous zest and pleasure.' In other words, not just regular exercise but a healthier diet, plenty of sleep and taking time to relax and visit friends. If we follow his advice we should be able to endure the stresses of modern life and still have energy left to enjoy recreation.

Pilates said, 'People won't understand the brilliance of my work for fifty years.' He was right. It is also reassuring to know that Joseph died aged eighty-seven and his wife Clara aged eighty. Both enjoyed good health (and looked amazing) into their old age.

Lynne Robinson

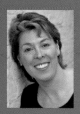

Instead of thinking of the last 28 days as a diet, we want you to think of them as a new healthy way of eating. Learning to listen to your body, changing the way you shop, the way you eat and the way you think about food will help change your habits and your attitude towards food which in turn will help you lose weight and stick to your new healthy regimen. Fruit and vegetables are a dieter's best friend – eating plenty of them is also one of the easiest routes to good health, so pile your plate high with fresh produce. Trim the fat by choosing low- and reduced-fat products whenever possible. Less fat doesn't have to mean less flavour and making small changes to your diet, such as switching to skimmed or semi-skimmed milk can make a real difference. Don't be afraid of eating carbohydrates, but do try to choose wholegrain varieties such as wholemeal bread and brown rice and learn to eat them in moderation. Make life easy for yourself – ensure your kitchen is well stocked with plenty of healthy foods and avoid buying those unhealthy foods you know you won't be able to resist.

Variety is the spice of life – it's also the key to a healthy diet, so don't get stuck in a food rut eating the same things week in week out. Introduce new foods into your diet and experiment with new recipes.

Being on a diet doesn't mean you have to forgo the pleasure of eating out, but learn to choose wisely from the menu avoiding anything fried or accompanied by a rich sauce. Don't devour the contents of the bread basket while you're waiting for your food to arrive – if you know you won't be able to resist picking at the bread, ask for it to be removed from the table. If you want something special don't be afraid to say that you would prefer your vegetables served without butter or your fish served without sauce, but make sure you do so when the waiter or waitress takes your order. Why not choose two starters rather than a starter and a main course, that way you won't feel too guilty if you want to finish your meal with something sweet. And don't feel you need to finish everything on your plate – learn to stop eating when you've had enough.

Finally, remember that good food is one of life's pleasures and choosing a healthy diet doesn't have to mean missing out on the foods you really enjoy – you simply need to learn to eat them in moderation.

Good luck – we know you can do it!

Fiona Hunter

# 6

## The Daily Workout Planner

We have given you five 30-minute workouts to do each week. You will need to have two days rest – either two consecutive days or two separate days, it doesn't matter which. What does matter, however, is that in addition you remember to do three 20-minute plus aerobic sessions each week. Choose the aerobic exercise from:

- brisk/power walking
- jogging
- swimming
- cycling
- rollerblading
- trampolining
- kick boxing
- spinning
- dancing
- skiing
- aerobics class
- cross-training
- rowing

Remind yourself of the general guidelines on pages 31–5.

These workouts have been designed to include all the main building blocks, so that at the end of the week you will have worked all the main muscle groups and completed a balanced fitness programme. For many of the exercises there are beginners, intermediate and advanced versions for you to choose from. You should obviously work at your level. If you have any injuries you should, of course, leave contraindicated exercises out.

Good luck and have fun!

Include the following exercises in your workout, choosing whichever level (beginners, intermediate, advanced) is appropriate:

## Apple Shape Workout

Spine Curls with Cushion 52
Studio Adductor Stretch 53
Curl Ups with Leg Extension 60
Oblique Curl Ups 61
Sitting Side Reach 80
Up and Down Barre Exercises 88
Arm Pulls 98
Standing Tarzan 97
Back Press with Weights 99
The Hundred 64
Double Leg Stretch 68
Hip Rolls 84
The Dart 74
The Star 75
Rest Position 79
The Torpedo 94
Side-lying Front and Back 92
Roll Downs with Weights 11

## Pear Shape Workout

Monkey Bends 86
Up and Down on One Leg 90
Demi-Pliés in Turn Out 87
Spine Curls with Cushion 52
Curl Ups with Leg Extension 60
Oblique Curl Ups 61
Single Leg Circles 56
The Hundred 64
Double Leg Stretch 68
Hip Rolls 84
Sitting Side Reach 80
The Torpedo 94
Side-lying Front and Back 92
Side-lying Bicycles 93
The Dart 74
Front Leg Pull 78
Rest Position 79
Arm Circles with Weights 95
Arm Weights: Triceps 96
Abductor Lifts 102
Inner Thigh Toner 104
Arm Openings 82

# Week One

## Workout One

## Workout Two

## Workout Three

## Workout Four

## Workout Five

# Week Two

## Workout One

## Workout Two

## Workout Three

## Workout Four

## Workout Five

# Week Three

## Workout One

## Workout Two

## Workout Three

## Workout Four

## Workout Five

# Week Four

## Workout One

Studio Adductor Stretch  53
Arm Openings  82
Single Leg Circles  56
Curl Ups  58
Demi-Pliés in Turn Out  87
The Hundred  64
Double Leg Stretch  68
The Diamond Press  72
The Star  75
Rest Position  79
Side-lying Front and Back  92
The Torpedo  94
Abductor Lifts  102
Inner Thigh Toner  104

## Workout Two

Spine Curls with Cushion  52
Sitting Twist  81
Curl Ups with Leg Extension  60
Oblique Curl Ups  61
Monkey Bends with Shoulder Reach  86
Double Leg Stretch  68
The Dart  74
Star Circles  77
Front Leg Pull  78
Rest Position  79
The Torpedo  94
Arm Circles with Weights  95
Arm Weights: Triceps  96
Roll Downs with Weights  100

## Workout Three

Beach Ball Hamstring Stretch  54
Pelvic Stability – Leg Slides, Drops,
   Folds and Turnout  44
Windows  55
Spine Curls with Cushion  52
Sitting Side Reach  80
Up and Down on One Leg  90
Kneeling Hip Flexor Stretch  85
The Hundred  64
Arm Openings  82
The Diamond Press  72
Rest Position  79
Abductor Lifts  102
Inner Thigh Toner  104

## Workout Four

Spine Curls with Cushion  52
Curl Ups  58
Single Leg Circles  56
Up and Down Barre Exercise  88
Arm Openings  82
Double Leg Stretch  68
The Dart  74
Rest Position  79
The Torpedo  94
Standing Tarzan  97
Arm Pulls  98
Back Press with Weights  99
Roll Downs with Weights  100

## Workout Five

The Starfish  50
Oblique Curl Ups  61
Studio Adductor Stretch  53
Sitting Side Reach  80
Hip Rolls  84
The Hundred  64
Double Leg Stretch  68
The Diamond Press  72
Front Leg Pull  78
The Star  75
Rest Position  79
Side-lying Front and Back  92
Side-lying Bicycles  93
Kneeling Hip Flexor Stretch  85
Arm Openings  82